Ferment Your Way to Good Health

Elisabeth Fekonia

Paperback: 978-1-966652-94-6
eBook: 978-1-966652-95-3
Library of Congress Control Number: 2025906793

This is a work of nonfiction.

Ordering Information:

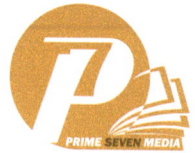

Prime Seven Media
518 Landmann St.
Tomah City, WI 54660

Printed in the United States of America

Table of Contents

Ferment your way to good health 1

Fermented Grains 9

Sourdough Bread 11
Sourdough Pikelets 16
Sourdough Pasta 17
Sourdough Wraps 18
Sourdough Pizza Base 19
Sourdough Crackers 20
Sourdough Slice 21
Fermented Banana Bread 22
Indian Steamed Bread Idli 23
Pancakes Made from Fermented Rice and Lentils – Dosa 24
Ogi 25
Fermented Polenta Fingers 26
Kishk: a breakfast cereal to serve with thin cream or milk 27
Soured Porridge Pot 28
Five Grain Cereal Mix 29
Five Grain Fermented Porridge 30
Ama Koji (a rice ferment) 31
Fermented Brown Rice 34

Fermented Legumes 35

Miso 37
How to make old-fashioned koji 38
Making the Miso 40
Tempeh 42
Fermented Bean Pate 44

Fermented Vegetables and Fruits 45

Fermented Apricot Spread 46
Fermented Raisin Chutney. 47
Fermented Pineapple/ Mango Chutney 48
Fermented Fruit Paste 49
Sauerkraut. 51
Kimchi 53
Cucumber Kimchi 54
Carrot kimchi. 55
Fermented Tomato Sauce 56
Nuka Doca 57

Fermented Dairy Products 59

Quark. 61
Neufchattel 62
Ricotta Cheese 63
Butter Kase (A German cheese meaning buttery cheese) 64
Feta 65
Brie Cheese 67
Camembert 68
Cheddar Cheese 69
Yoghurt 71
Kefir. 73
Cultured Butter 76

Fermented Beverages 78

Fermented Rice Milk 80
Rejuvelac 81
Ginger Beer 82
Lactic Fermented Ginger Ale 84
Water Kefir. 85
Orange-Ginger Carrot Kvass 87
Lactic-Fermented Sweet Potato Fly 88
Kombucha Tea 89
Beet Kvass 91

Ferment your way to good health

What are fermented foods?

In days of old people knew how to extend the life of their food without the advantage of our modern storage methods. Organisms were employed to do the job of preserving or pickling foods and beverages. These organisms consist of certain types of bacteria, moulds or fungi or a combination of these. Most ferments are made with lactic-forming bacteria, and this will give the food a slightly sour taste. Other foods such as miso, soy sauce and tempeh are mould-based ferments, and fermented tea or kombucha is an example of a fungi- or mushroom-based ferment.

Health benefits of fermented foods

Adding fermented food to your daily diet is considered one way of preventing disease. These powerhouse foods will help to eliminate inflammation, which is the cause behind many illnesses such as cancer and heart disease, excess cholesterol and Alzheimer's. Eliminate inflammation and you will cut down the risk of disease. Modern research shows that beneficial bacteria, otherwise known as probiotics (the opposite of antibiotics), help balance the gut flora in your digestive system and reduce the levels of toxic pathogens that cause ill health. Other research also suggests that the regular consumption of live lactobacilli bacteria can improve your gut flora and reduce the number of infections by reducing pathogens.

Fermented foods enhance digestion

There are many digestive enzymes found in fermented foods, and these will spare your own enzymes. Enzymes will aid digestion, increase vitamin levels, are bowel cleansing, and result in the general improvement in our good health. Many people suffer toxicity from stress, exposure to chemicals and pollutants from the environment and/or a poor diet. All these factors affect our gut and digestive health, and these live probiotic foods are the first line of defence to build up a healthy immune system. Allergies can also be corrected with these probiotics; they can also help to prevent migraines, lethargy, or just feeling tired. Fermentation breaks down the nutrients in foods by the action of beneficial microorganisms and creates natural chelators that are available to bind toxins and remove them from the body.

Some examples of fermented foods

Sourdough bread, cheese and cultured foods such as sauerkraut, kimchi, miso, tempeh, soy sauce and wine are but a few examples of fermented foods and beverages. As you can see in this book from the many and varied types of ferments that are available, any food or drink can be fermented and there's nothing to stop you from experimenting and creating your own. In times of old before the industrial age, people naturally knew to ferment a proportion of their food and drinks to enhance flavour, extend the life of their foods, and for a general feeling of good health. Since modern-day food storage, the old ways have been largely forgotten but in recent times a huge revival is taking place, and many people are waking up to the taste and health benefits of fermented foods. I can't imagine a day going by without eating or drinking something fermented as it keeps me feeling 'just right'. I would really miss it after a few days of going without, so watch out – fermented food can become addictive!

Where to get fermented foods

Unfortunately, live fermented foods are very hard to find in retail outlets, the exception being kimchi which can be found in Asian supermarkets. Coconut yoghurt is another example, but some contain too much sugar. Sauerkraut is mostly pasteurised unless you can find the organic varieties, and a lot of sourdough breads are not true sourdoughs either. The fermentation process involves time, and the manufacturer always looks for shortcuts to reduce overheads and consequently there are many fake fermented foods around.

I think you may be concluding that fermented foods and beverages need to be made by you, at home, in your own kitchen. This is not necessarily a scary thing, although often newcomers to fermentation are rather worried of getting it wrong and think they may make their friends and family sick with their fermenting efforts. The reason for this fear is understandable as leaving food at room temperature to ferment instead of keeping it cold in the fridge for safe keeping, seems like a very contradictory thing to do. Therefore, the purpose of this book is to demystify the art of fermentation, so you the reader, will have a greater understanding of how it all works and that you won't be afraid of doing it for yourself.

Safety aspect of fermented food

I am often asked how can you be sure that fermented foods are safe to eat? This question is easily answered. No matter how civilised we deem ourselves to be, we still have that inherent little voice inside us that will tell us if something smells and tastes healthy or not. So do trust your instinct. Fermented foods have their own aroma and though they may smell unfamiliar to you, you can still tell if that smell is healthy or not. I recommend you make it a habit to smell and taste any fermented food you come across to become familiar with how they should smell.

Acidity is what keeps food safe – just like with making traditional chutneys and relishes, the presence of vinegar creates an acidic environment that keeps the pickled food from spoiling. Lactic fermentation also creates an acidic environment, hence the slightly sour taste, but lactic fermentation does more than keep the food intact and safe to eat. It enhances digestion as the food is pre-digested by the action of all these organisms. Chutneys and relishes do nothing to help digest our food – food boiled in sugar and vinegar is meant to preserve the food and contribute to taste but nothing more.

Many fermented foods are based on lactic fermentation, and this is created by lactic-forming bacteria that creates its own low pH. Acidity does not give the food-spoilage bacteria a toehold to spoil the food as they require an alkaline environment to do their job of decomposition. Therefore, if a lactic fermented food loses its acidity and becomes bland in taste, it's time to throw it into the compost bin.

More on the health benefits of fermented food: Your health is your wealth

There is a saying that your food should be your medicine and that you are what you eat. There is a lot of truth in this and the food you eat certainly influences your general well-being. Are you getting everything you need to give you abundance of good health or do you feel that your diet is somehow letting you down? There are many foods that we can eat that will greatly enhance digestion and nutrient uptake. It is important to look at how we digest and assimilate our food, as this is where trouble often starts. Older people have fewer digestive enzymes than younger people, as we tend to lose our storehouse of enzymes with every passing year. Live, raw, fermented foods enhance the digestion of the entire meal. The following suggestions are helpful hints to regain health and vitality simply by eating foods that are your medicine.

The digestive process

It all starts with a desire to eat. You can smell the food being prepared and you are getting hungry. Your stomach juices signal you for action and you look forward to tucking into it. When you are chewing your food, the digestive processes have well and truly started. Food needs to be chewed thoroughly and then it will be digested where the stomach is ready and waiting with all those digestive juices ready for action. This is the first important hint for good health. Ingesting some lactic fermented food will also stimulate the salivary glands that will in turn start the digestive juices flowing in the stomach.

A good balance of gut bacteria and digestive enzymes helps you to absorb more of the nutrients from the food you eat. You are what you assimilate, not what you eat! You won't need as many supplements as you'll be absorbing more from live foods.

A lot of people suffer from a low pH (acidity) and this is where trouble gets a foothold. With a low pH, arthritis and other degenerative diseases do their damage to joints and blood vessels. Our ideal pH is slightly alkaline – 7.3 to 7.4, and you can test your own pH by using a simple soil test kit by testing your saliva or urine. How do you change a pH that is too acidic? By eating lots of fresh greens and fruit and vegetables will automatically readjust a pH that is out of kilter. Drinking fresh carrot and celery juice will also go a long way to good health. A glass of lemon juice or a dash of raw apple cider vinegar is an excellent way to start the day. Also, a small glass of kefir fizzy fruit drink will help to adjust your pH to a more alkaline state as well as a glass of kombucha tea.

How do fermented foods work for us?

Fermentation is the art of breaking down complex starches to simpler sugars, proteins into amino acids, and sugars into lactic acid by using specific microbes. Fermentation also creates digestive enzymes, vitamins and many other compounds that contribute to more efficient nutrient absorption.

People consuming a wholemeal diet without any fermented food will tend to have mineral deficiencies as well as impeded digestive systems. This is due to the phytic acid and enzyme inhibitors that are bound in the outer layer of the bran. They are present in all grains, legumes, nuts and seeds. These will play havoc with digestion and contribute to dental caries if they aren't neutralized by soaking, sprouting or fermenting.

Enzyme inhibitors are an important force in the life of grains, legumes, nuts and seeds, as they are all effectively seeds waiting to germinate into new plants. These inhibitors are there to keep the seed intact until germination is ensured as their genetics will then be passed onto the next generation. These irritating factors are neutralized when the seed sprouts into new life, soaking and fermentation will have the same effect.

Conventional bread-baker's yeast cannot be compared with the natural leavening process of sourdough. It does nothing to improve the bread except to make it taste nice and have an airy texture. The whole meal bread will have the effect of inhibiting our own digestive enzymes due to the phytic acid found in the bran, and this will impede the proper absorption of minerals such as calcium, iron, magnesium and zinc. Fermentation such as the old-fashioned leavening process of sourdough will neutralize these mineral and enzyme inhibitors. This makes the food much better for your health and tastier for you to enjoy.

A diet rich in fermented foods also encourages healthy gut flora and this is of utmost importance to our good health. Apparently, no cancer patient has good gut flora. The bowel can be the seat of disease.

Are there any other foods that will help with our digestion?

Spices such as galangal, ginger and turmeric are excellent, and these can easily be incorporated into the dishes we prepare. Eating lots of garlic, onions, leeks and fibre rich foods will also help with our well-being. These foods are called prebiotics, and they help the friendly bacteria to flourish in a clean environment. Some people feel that food combining works for them and this means that starches and proteins aren't eaten together at the same meal. If we have a good intake of digestive enzymes, this might not be so important.

Are you getting all your minerals?

Today's food is falling far short of being nutrient dense. Soils are generally mineral deficient due to constant chemical applications, and you can't expect to have all your mineral needs met. Soil needs to be rich in organic matter and teeming with life to grow healthy wholesome food.

No wonder there are so many people in our society that have digestive problems!

Become mineral saturated and attain good energy levels by supplementing with a plant-based mineral supplement until you can adjust your diet to an organic one. Celtic sea salt is also an excellent way of getting a lot of minerals into your diet. Don't be afraid to enjoy using this salt. use it freely to make food taste great as well as help to saturate yourself with up to eighty different minerals from the sea. Using this salt (as well as Himalayan and pink lake salt) will not raise your blood pressure; in fact, it could help to lower it! Plants, animals, people and soil that have their full quota of minerals generally don't get sick

Natural antibiotics

There are foods that have a special quality within them, and they act as natural antibiotics. Mould on sourdough bread has special qualities that will help to combat pathogens. Consuming tempeh will also provide a heat-resistant natural antibiotic for optimal health. Brie and Camembert have natural antibiotic properties as well.

Another source of a natural antibiotic is colloidal silver. Colloidal silver is also antifungal and antiviral and is very useful as a first defense against oncoming colds, flu and toothache. High doses of vitamin C are also recommended. This is best taken in a powder form as vitamin C tablets often have saccharin in them.

Probiotics

It is so important to have a healthy population of gut flora. Modern-day living with stress, pollution, antibiotics and other medication will upset the balance of the beneficial bacteria required for the proper digestion and nutrient assimilation of our food. These naturally occurring bowel flora need to be included in the diet to maintain a healthy population. This will help enhance the immune system as well as create more vitamins and complete the breaking down process.

The flora in milk and water kefir will be killed off as it moves through the digestive process, but the upper intestinal tract will have the benefits of balancing the pH to where it's needed in the right places for optimum digestion. The kefir organisms will also increase peristaltic action as they move food down through the gut. Lactic ferments will help greatly towards building a healthy environment within the digestive tract, and a wide variety of fermented foods with their own organisms will also bring a great storehouse of many types of life to build up a healthy immune system. Such an environment will give the biggest protection against cancer as this disease won't get a toehold with all those friendly bacteria standing guard.

Prebiotics

Providing food for the good bugs comes in the form of prebiotics. These are composed of the allum family, onions, leeks, garlic. Bitter greens such as chicory, radicchio and dandelion leaves as well as Jerusalem artichokes, yacon, and cocao and flaxseeds are among other plants that provide fibre we don't digest but feed the friendly bacteria that reside in our large colon. Green bananas or plantains are full of resistant starches that our friendly gut bacteria love to feed on and help overcome the bad guys.

Natural cleansers

Sometimes when the body feels sluggish or you don't feel quite well, it would be a good idea to have a cleanup. Liken it to a good spring clean where debris that clogs up the system needs to be removed and washed out. The most effective way is to embark on a juice fast for several days where the digestive process has a break from digesting food. This gives the body a chance to do its own repairs. A diet high in fibre is also like a natural cleanser and glucuronic acid occurs naturally in the liver and is also produced by the mushroom tea, kombucha. Kombucha is a very pleasant, slightly acidic and fizzy tea and drinking it will aid and cleanse the liver. It is also advisable to drink lots of water during the day but make sure it is pure, clean, filtered rain or spring water.

Last of all, remember to get rid of the chemicals in your life. We are living in a very toxic age, and this contributes to many forms of cancer. Eating lots of beans will help rid the body of heavy metals but remember to soak them in water with some kefir water before cooking. Also remember that soybeans should always be traditionally fermented first and eaten with discretion.

Our unseen friends

Many people are afraid to leave food out on the bench to grow these organisms to ferment their food. It is so contrary to what we have been taught, as we have always put food in the fridge to keep it from going off. Storing our food in the fridge will greatly reduce the food spoilage bacteria from ruining the food simply by keeping the food at a very cool temperature, fermenting food on the other hand is doing the opposite – we leave food out at ambient room temperature to grow bacteria, enzymes, moulds and yeasts to pickle or ferment the food.

Everything will ferment faster on a hot summer's day as opposed to a slower result on a cold winter's day, so the timing of fermenting will need to be adjusted. Fermentation is about giving the food a controlled environment and that is usually done by introducing the right organisms to grow and proliferate in that food. A lot of fermentation is done by immersing the food under liquid, be it under its own juices or simply under water with the addition of the right bacteria and some salt. Most fermentation is classed as wild, as organisms are easily captured from the air around us.

We take in many different types of bacteria – as we breathe the air and with every bite we take, bacteria are always entering our bodies as that is how we have been designed. We need these organisms, and we have developed specialised strategies to keep pathogens under control by having good gut health. In contrast to what we have been taught, we don't need to kill all the germs to be in good health. In fact, we need lots of them to stay healthy! If we keep the troublemakers in smaller numbers, we will have what is called homeostasis as our intestinal flora will then be in balance. Our good health depends on a greater number of friendly bacteria and a much smaller number of pathogens.

The human body is home to millions of beneficial bacteria. In fact, the average healthy human has around one to two kilos of these organisms! We house millions of bacteria on our skin and in our nose, mouth and gut. We wouldn't be able to survive without bacteria. We are born sterile but during the natural birth passage we ingest our mother's gut flora and inoculate our own gut for the rest of our lives. Bacteria help us to stay in good health. Antibiotics on the other hand can wipe out our body's beneficial bacteria, causing unwanted health consequences. This competitive effect becomes apparent when we wipe out a large proportion of our intestinal flora, for instance by an antibiotic that is prescribed to treat a bacterial infection. Diarrhoea is frequently the unwanted result, as 'foreign' bacteria take their chance to occupy the empty niches. Healthy bacteria will take over in time, so that in most cases the side effects of antibiotics will wear off but that can take as long as two years.

It is recommended though, that to get the balance of friendly bacteria back in their maximum numbers again, we should consume prebiotic and probiotic foods and beverages. There are far too many factors in our lives that may prevent us from getting our friendly bacteria population back in the required numbers without some assistance; the toxic environment we live in, unrelenting stress, eating on the run and junk food will all hamper the building up of these naturally occurring bacteria.

Preparing for fermentation

To make sure that the right bacteria and organisms are growing in the food that we are preparing for fermentation, we need to inoculate them with some starter cultures. These cultures are found in nature, and we use them as a kind of insurance policy so that the ferment will get off to a good start. Lactic-forming bacteria are everywhere, and this is why lactic fermentation is the most popular of all ferments. These organisms are found on the leaves of plants, on our skin and in the air. We also find them in kefir, juice, sauerkraut and kimchi liquid, and on the skins of fruit and vegetables.

Pathogens can't thrive in an acidic environment, but the right organisms do. Using some sea salt at the start of a new ferment inhibits putrefaction bacteria; only a little is needed as the lactic-forming bacteria will kick in in enough numbers after the first few days to take over the preservation of the food. Using more salt, such as 1–1½ tablespoons per litre hardens the pectin in the vegetables, leaving them crunchy and enhancing the flavour. The more salt that is used, the slower the fermentation process and the saltier the final taste. If no salt is used, then the ferment will turn out mushy and that is not desirable either so a balance of flavour and texture needs to be explored to determine how much salt you will need to use for a ferment that is to your liking.

The inoculants

Milk and water kefir are very useful for introducing a great number of lactic-forming bacteria into a new batch of food or beverage for fermenting.

There are other types of inoculants to use to start a new ferment. Sour whey from yoghurt and kefir milk, kombucha tea (not on its own though), and sauerkraut juice can also be used as a starter as well as rejuvelac. These all contain a host of lactic bacteria and other organisms that are suitable as a starter.

Fermented Grains

Grains are hard on our digestive systems, and it's been said that we don't digest any grain completely. Undigested particles of grain get stuck in the microvilli of our intestinal walls, building up with time, and ultimately undermining our ability to properly digest other foods. Gluten is a very difficult-to-digest protein, and it puts a tremendous strain on the digestive system, and with age, allergies, celiac disease, mental illness, chronic indigestion, and candida overgrowth can result. Gluten intolerance has also been associated with multiple sclerosis.

Moreover, we must battle with phytic acid and antinutrients that are present in whole meal grains as they lock up minerals and enzymes. When phytic acid gets loose in our own guts, it binds with the vitamins and minerals and keeps us from absorbing them. This can lead to a host of systemic problems, most notably dental decay.

It turns out that traditional grain preparation techniques solve these problems.

Let's take a few samples of food to see the varying phytic acid levels found in them:

(In milligrams per 100 grams of dry weight)

Brazil nuts	1,719	Cocoa powder	1,684–1,796	Brown rice	12,509
Oat flakes	1,174	Walnuts	982	Raw peanuts	821
Lentils	779	Hazel nuts	648–1000	Corn	367
White flour	268	White rice	11.5–66.0		

Traditional grain preparation includes soaking in an acidic medium such as the addition of sour whey in the soaking water, or by sourdough fermentation. Some traditional societies soak their grains for up to several days to ensure the breakdown of all the nasties. In India, rice and lentils are fermented for at least two days before being made into idli and dosa; in Scotland, oats are soaked overnight before being cooked into porridge; Mexicans soak their corn for several days before making their corn bread cakes. The early pioneers of America always kept back some of their sourdough for the next batch.

A loaf of bread you buy today will be full of additives such as mould inhibitors, dough conditioners, preservatives and in some cases sugar along with pesticide residues and gluten. If the bread is whole meal, it will have phytates, and enzyme inhibitors as well. We can't call this bread the 'staff of life' anymore – bread today has become like junk food to our bodies. New flour hybrids bred for today's bread also have a higher gluten content for a lighter, airier texture but we pay the price for it with our health.

You can see now that in our modern society, wheat and grain products have not been treated in the time-honoured way. In the last few generations, modern food processing methods have taken food production out of our hands. Food is seen purely as a commodity with little consideration given to its nutritional content. Until a few generations ago when people still baked their own bread, they knew about the powers of fermentation on grains. It was passed down from one generation to the next. In fact, some sourdough starters were several generations old! Unfortunately, we lost these skills, and we are only just reviving them with the new interest in growing and producing real food. Yes, we are turning full circle, and we are sure to pick up the many benefits of our recaptured knowledge of fermented foods.

Sourdough Bread

Sourdough is the old-fashioned way of making bread and it's making a great comeback. It is a natural leavening that changes the chemistry within the dough: complex starches turn into simple sugars, enzyme inhibitors and phytates are neutralized out, and the gluten is broken down to the point where there is only a limited rise left in the dough. It is for this reason that many people who are sensitive to gluten or who are gluten intolerant can freely enjoy sourdough without any ill effects. A lot of people over the years have told me they can eat bread again due to the natural breaking down of the gluten in sourdough.

With this kind of ferment, the bread will be much easier to digest, and it will be tastier as well.

Making sourdough is a totally natural experience from beginning to end and with this fact in mind, the variations in taste will reflect your own immediate environment. Just like with cheese making and any other natural ferments, moulds and yeasts that inhabit the food preparation area will all be reflected in the sourdough starter that you make.

The starter

Sourdough bread needs a starter to ferment. To make a starter all you need to do is to add equal amounts of water with flour and leave it in a warm spot to ferment. It's as simple as that. However, there are factors that can influence this process and these are as follows:

- Freshly ground organic flour will give optimum results but any flour that doesn't have preservatives and has been bleached will be fine too.
- Temperature is an influence but is not important. The warmer the conditions the quicker the yeasts will grow and multiply. Cooler temperatures will retard but not stop the process. (You can make sourdough in the fridge for instance.)

- The mixture should be fluid enough for the yeasts to grow and thrive. An improvement to this simple mixture would be to add a little sour whey/ water kefir, to introduce some more yeasts, bacteria and enzymes to give it a start. This will help to make a more effective starter culture.

My own sourdough starter mixture consists of two ingredients:

½ cup of unbleached flour

water

(optional) ½ cup of water/ milk kefir, yoghurt or buttermilk

1. Mix the ingredients together into a thin cream consistency adjusting the liquid as needed and place in a bowl with a tea towel or some open-weave cloth to keep any insects out but still have contact with the air.

2. Stir daily and it should be ready in about a week in the summer and about ten days to two weeks in the cooler weather. On stirring you will soon see some little bubbles and froth with a faint yeasty aroma that will come from the mixture. Don't be in a hurry but look for signs of activity. No need to feed this starter as there's plenty of food for the small population of microbes.

Whenever a starter has been sitting in the fridge for over six weeks, it's best to refresh the starter a day or so before bread-making day. Simply add some fresh flour and water and leave out of the fridge overnight. This will give all those hungry little organisms the fresh food they are starving for.

There are many other recipes that will give you a sourdough starter such as fermented apple juice mixed with flour, or by using mashed potato. These different starter cultures might make a slight change in taste in the sourdough bread, but after using your starter for a while, the yeasts and other microorganisms that are in the air in your kitchen will alter their characteristics back to your own environment. Isn't it wonderful to experience the natural forces at work?

Oh, one more thing about starters, and it makes me cringe when I hear of a starter that has been passed down for many generations! It is nothing special, believe me. It just shows that some people have been making sourdough bread for generations, but the starter is not precious at all. I would easily make another starter if I had an accident with mine and lost it.

The sponge

The sponge is the preparation for making the sourdough bread and it is also the first rising. The consistency of a sponge is in between a dough and a batter, and the yeasts will have a better chance to work in a more liquid environment.

The second rising can only occur by the off gassing of the organisms during the feeding process. The following day you will be feeding the organisms in the sponge by adding more flour to turn it into a dough ready for the second rising in the bread tins.

1. Start with a large bowl and place some starter culture in it. (quarter to half a cup is ample for a runny starter) A dough starter will only need about a tablespoon of starter dough.

2. Add some water to dissolve it and then add the flour, some salt, and any other ingredients that you might care to add. (See suggestions below.)

3. It is very difficult to give measurements as different types of flour will absorb differing amounts of water. As a rule of thumb use three cups of flour to mix up the sponge and reserve the fourth cup to knead the sponge into a dough the next day.

After mixing the water into the flour, give the bowl a shake and see if the whole lot wobbles. This is called the wobble test. If it doesn't wobble, add more water to make it more like a soft sponge. As you can see this is very technical!

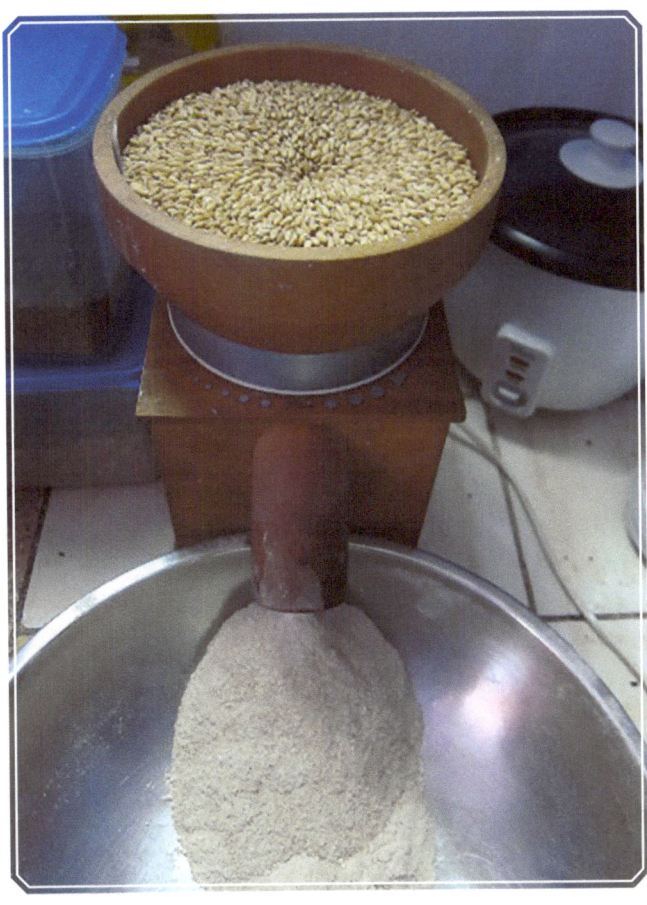

Freshly ground, organic flour made with a flour grinder.

Extra Ingredients:

There is so much you can add to your bread to give it extra taste, texture and nutritional content. I always feel it's important for my daily bread to be the staff-of-life bread, just like bread used to be. Value adding as suggested below will truly make your sourdough the best it can be.

Kelp	Sunflower seed
Carob or cacao	Dried fruits
Flaxseed oil	Herbs
Linseed	Spices
Pumpkin seed	

I recommend adding carob or cacao powder – not only does it make it look dark like a rye bread, but it gives antioxidants and various other health benefits.

Anything else you wish to add is up to you. I often grind some linseed in a coffee grinder and throw in some whole seed as well.

I also use some sweet whey instead of water if I have been making cheese. Not only will it give more nutrition but it will create a stronger bread with the extra proteins from the whey. If you would like to add other types of flour into the bread mix you will need to keep in mind that the loaf will turn out a lot denser and heavier. Rye and barley flour will have less gluten than wheat, and other grains will have none. I suggest you try making sourdough with wheat first before attempting to use other grains. Oh, and don't forget to add some salt.

Be sure to wait until the fermentation process is complete and the mixture should look and smell alive with bubbles and air pockets.

The next morning add enough flour in the bowl to turn the sponge into a dough. Remember this extra flour will be food for all the microorganisms that have been multiplying in the sponge overnight. The second rising will now be much quicker, and this will only take a few hours. Wait until the loaf has doubled in size before baking.

Butter your bread tins generously for a nice crusty loaf and take enough dough to half fill a tin. Knead, adding flour as required to keep the dough from sticking to the bench. Take care not to add too much flour or the result will be a dry and boring bread. Aim for flour saturation, i.e. add just enough to prevent the dough from sticking to the bench, and you will soon be able to knead the dough without adding more. Keep the bench and your hands clean so you can gauge when you get to that flour saturation point. I find that twelve times kneading of the dough without having to add flour to prevent it from sticking, is a good indication that the dough is ready for the second rising. Any more flour added after this will result in a dry bread that is not very interesting to eat and only toasting will save it.

Place the kneaded dough in the bread tins and allow to rise till double in size. This should be enough to give a nice, rounded top after the bread has risen. Be careful not to underfill or overfill the bread tins as a small loaf will give you very short slices and get lost in the toaster, and if too much dough is placed in the pan, there will be a messy overflow in the rising process. Allow the bread tins to sit undisturbed with a tea towel over them until the loaves have risen enough to give them a slightly rounded top. This will take a few hours in hot weather and the best part of the day in cold weather.

Have a pre-heated oven ready at 210°C. Take the tins to the oven taking care not to bump them as they can collapse. Bake for 45 minutes and the bread will look baked and have that hollow sound when tapped on the bottom. The sides should be firm to the touch and not feel doughy when pressed and the colour should be just coming onto a golden brown. Your temperature and timing may need adjusting depending on the efficiency of your oven.

N.B. Use the smaller size bread pans as the larger ones tend to undercook the bread inside. Sourdough is denser than conventional bread due to the breaking down of the gluten.

The bread you make will be unlike any other, as the organisms in your kitchen environment are unique to your surroundings!

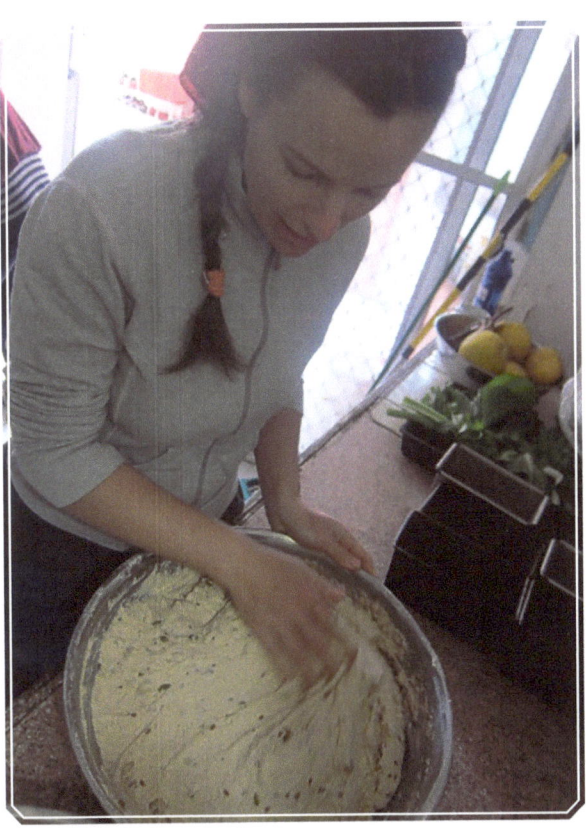

Sourdough Pikelets

1. Mix a bit of starter (quarter of a cup is ample) in some water and dissolve it

2. Add enough flour and some salt to make up a sponge and allow to ferment overnight

3. Take about 2½–3 cups of sourdough sponge and add 1 egg. (I always reserve some of the sourdough sponge in a separate bowl. This is to make sure that if the mixture accidentally becomes too liquid then there will be enough of the sponge mixture to add to the pikelet mix as adding flour at this stage will ruin the taste.) Add enough water to allow the batter to drop off a dessertspoon making sure it doesn't become too runny

4. When the consistency is just right, add ½ teaspoon of bicarbonate of soda. Allow the mixture to froth and bubble

5. Have a medium hot frying pan ready and place some ghee or coconut oil in the pan. Carefully spoon the pikelet mix into the frying pan allowing plenty of space for expansion. Flip over and cook on the other side

These pikelets are best eaten fresh while they are still warm. They have their own sweetness because of the fermentation so there is no need to add any sugar. The flour's complex starches have been transformed into simpler sugars, making them guilt-free.

Variation: You can also turn these pikelets into pancakes by making them larger in size. By omitting the bicarb of soda and adding more milk or water, you can also make paper thin crepes.

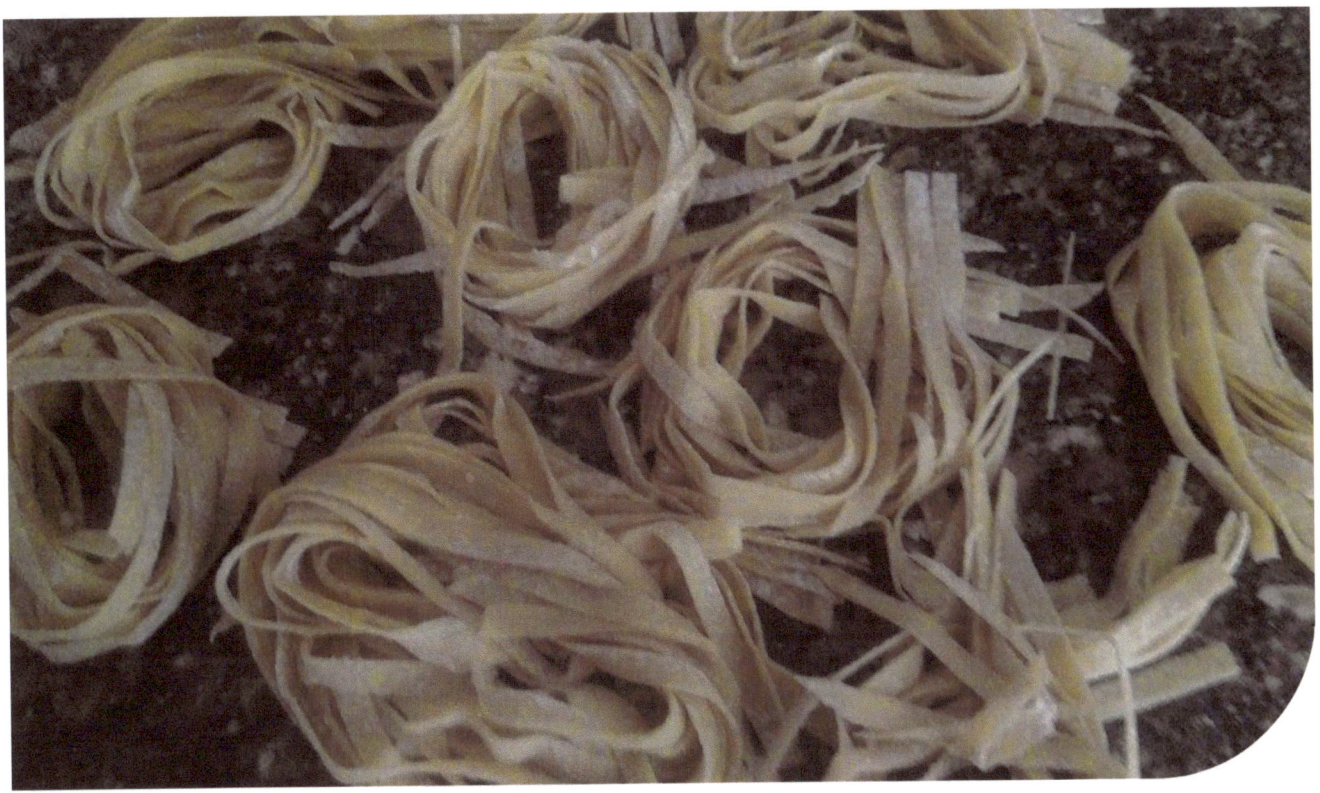

Sourdough Pasta

2 cups hard wheat flour
(I use high gluten white flour)

3 eggs

Salt

¼ cup runny sourdough starter

1. Combine all the ingredients into a dough and allow to rise in a covered bowl overnight

2. The next morning add more flour if necessary until it creates deep folds in the dough. It will take a bit of kneading, but it will come smooth and elastic after a while

3. Allow to do a second rise in time for making pasta for lunch or dinner time

4. Sprinkle tapioca flour on the bench and roll out the dough quite thin. If you have a pasta maker, then proceed to roll out your small amounts of pasta dough instead of manually rolling it out with a rolling pin. You can then make the cuts for the strands and pile them on a plate. Have a pot of boiling water ready and throw all the pasta strands in at once and separate the hot strands with a pasta server so it all comes loose on impact of the boiling water. The pasta can also be rolled into tagliatelle strands then dried on a tray for about 24 hours. When the pasta is bone dry it can be stored in a container for up to two months on your pantry shelf in an airtight container.

Sourdough Wraps

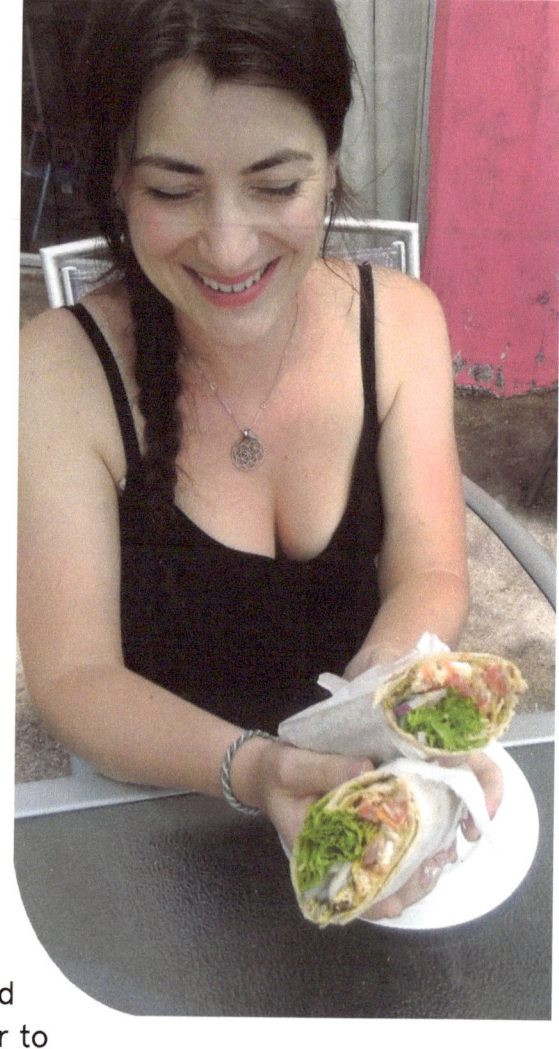

Two cups of white high gluten flour (double 0)

Any spices of your choice (Herb and garlic seasoning works well)

3 eggs

2 dessert spoons liquid coconut oil

¼ cup runny sourdough starter

1 teaspoon salt

1. In the evening place all the ingredients in a bowl and mix into a dough

2. The next morning add more flour if needed and around lunch time add some tapioca flour to achieve the right firmness in the dough to roll out into wraps

3. Have a very hot dry frying pan ready and cook quickly on both sides

4. The dough will keep in the fridge for around 6 weeks. Just take off about 90 grams of dough to roll out and bake into a wrap as you need them. This batch will make 5 wraps

Sourdough Pizza Base

Makes two standard pizza bases

1 cup white and 1 cup wholemeal flour

½ cup runny sourdough starter

¾ cup water

1 tablespoon olive oil

1 teaspoon salt

1. Mix the sourdough starter, olive oil, the salt to 1 ¼ cups of flour. Add more flour, a little at a time, as needed to form a pizza dough consistency. The amount of flour needed will depend on the hydration level of your sourdough starter
2. Allow the dough to ferment overnight
3. Next morning knead the dough and add some more flour if necessary to achieve a reasonable firmness and allow to rise for a few hours
4. Roll out the dough onto two pizza trays and prick the base with a fork
5. Bake the pizza base for approximately 7 minutes
6. Add the desired toppings and bake the pizza until the crust browns and the cheese melts

Freezing Pizza Dough

You can freeze pizza dough before rolling them out into rounds. Cover the dough with a coating of oil and seal airtight in plastic freezer bags. They will keep in good condition for around 3 months in the freezer. Defrost in the fridge before taking it out to come to room temperature before rolling out.

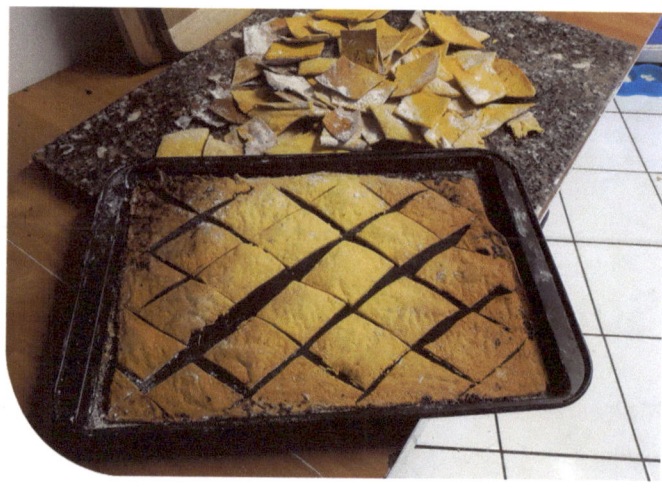

Sourdough Crackers

These crackers have become a huge hit in workshops whenever I present them with the homemade cheese

2½ cups high gluten white flour (Italian flour)

1 cup runny sourdough starter

4 tablespoons olive oil

Italian mixed herbs /barbeque spice mix/ smokey paprika

sea salt

1. In a bowl mix the spices into the flour

2. Add the runny sourdough starter and olive oil and mix thoroughly with a spoon

3. Knead it all together in the bowl, perhaps adding a few tablespoons of runny starter to have the dough just moist enough to come together if its still a little dry

4. Leave the dough at room temperature overnight

5. The next day divide the dough into portions. Roll them out with some tapioca starch to avoid adding more gluten and place the thin dough on a dry baking tray by unrolling from the rolling pin

6. Sprinkle some salt over the dough and lightly press it in. Sesame seeds, or any other topping of choice can be added for interest

7. Cut the dough diagonally into diamonds

8. Bake for approximately 15 minutes or until just golden brown in a moderate oven

Sourdough Slice

1 cup runny sourdough starter

3 cups flour

1 teaspoon bicarb of soda

¼ cup butter

¼ cup coconut oil

1 cup rapadura/ coconut sugar

1 egg

1 tsp. vanilla extract

½ teaspoon salt

Choc chips (optional but nice)

1. Cream together butter, coconut oil and egg in a food processor
2. Mix in the sourdough starter and vanilla extract
3. In a separate bowl, combine the dry ingredients
4. Mix the wet and dry ingredients together and press into a greased tray and finish with a fork making it smooth all over
5. Allow the dough to ferment overnight
6. Bake for 15 to 20 minutes in a moderate oven or until done

Fermented Banana Bread

3 cups flour

2 cups buttermilk, soured raw milk, or 2 cups of water with 2 tablespoons sour whey, yoghurt or water kefir

3 eggs, lightly beaten

1 teaspoon sea salt

¼ to ½ cup maple syrup/honey or ama koji

2 teaspoons bicarb of soda

¼ cup melted butter

2 ripe bananas, mashed

1. Mix the flour with the buttermilk and stand to ferment overnight

2. Beat in the remaining ingredients and pour into a well buttered and floured loaf tin

3. Bake in a moderate oven for one hour or until a toothpick comes out clean

Indian Steamed Bread Idli

2 cups of glutinous or medium grain white rice

1 cup of lentils (red lentils make a lovely pink batter)

1 cup of yoghurt or kefired milk or kefired coconut milk

1 teaspoon bicarbonate of soda

1 teaspoon salt

1. Soak both the rice and lentils together in a bowl overnight

2. Strain the water off the next day

3. Place in a food processor and whiz until it becomes a fine mush. The batter should be near pouring consistency

4. Add the yoghurt or kefir and leave to ferment for 24 to 48 hours (depending on ambient temperature)

5. Once it has risen substantially, add the salt and bicarb of soda and pour into a container that will fit into a steamer

6. Steam until firm to touch

Pancakes Made from Fermented Rice and Lentils – Dosa

Use the same ingredients as for the Indian steamed bread.

1. When the batter has fermented, add 1 cup of lukewarm water to thin the batter
2. Add seasoning such as chopped parsley/ coriander and grated ginger
3. Heat a well-seasoned frying pan with ghee and use a ladle to pour some batter into the centre of the frying pan using a spiralling motion
4. Flip over to the other side just like a pancake when bubbles appear on the surface
5. Stuff the dosa with savoury fillings and roll up and serve with yoghurt or kefir

Ogi

A fermented cereal porridge from West Africa, typically made from maize, sorghum, or millet. Traditionally, the grains are soaked in water for up to three days, before wet milling and sieving to remove husks. The filtered cereal is then allowed to ferment for up to three days until sour. It is then boiled into a pap, or cooked to make a stiff porridge. The fermentation of Ogi is performed by various lactic acid bacteria and various yeasts including Saccharomyces

1 cup of millet

5 ½ cups water

¼ cup sour whey/water kefir

1. Place the millet in a bowl, cover with 2 cups of water and leave to soak for 24 hours

2. Pour off the excess water and put through the food processor to grind it into a paste

3. Pour the slurry into a cloth lined strainer and pour 1 cup of water through the slurry into a bowl underneath the strainer. Discard the slurry when all the water has passed through. Add the sour whey/ Kefir to the resulting liquid and allow to ferment for 24 to 72 hours depending on room temperature. Stir daily

4. Add the remaining 2 ½ cups of water and now this liquid can now be boiled into a porridge. Cook gently stirring frequently. This porridge can be quite sour in taste, but it is oh-so-delicious with the addition of some coconut or rapadura sugar

Fermented Polenta Fingers

Polenta is a firm favourite with Italian people but fermenting the cornmeal is virtually unknown in their cuisine. Fermenting doesn't only get rid of the phytic acid; it enhances the flavour and increases its browning properties so the polenta fingers can be fried in hot ghee or coconut oil for a delicious accompaniment to any meal.

250 g of maize meal or polenta and two tablespoons sour whey/ water kefir

1. Soak the polenta in a bowl with a generous amount of water and sour whey. Leave to ferment for several days then pour off the excess water (I give the soaking water to my livestock because the lactic bacteria will benefit their gut flora or save the fermenting water as a starter to initiate new ferments)

2. Add enough water to the pan to make the fermented polenta swim a little and add some salt to taste

3. Cook it up into a very thick porridge until the whole mass leaves the sides of the pan and it can't be stirred or cooked anymore without burning

4. Pour the contents onto a clean marble slab and form into a neat rectangle of about 1 ½ centimetres thick. Make sure to neaten the edges as much as possible – you can use the wooden spoon to do this

5. When the slab has cooled down, cut it into fingers with a sharp knife. Lift the pieces into a container with a lid to prevent them from drying out, and keep in the fridge until needed

6. Heat a frying pan with some ghee and fry on both sides until just golden brown. This makes an excellent accompaniment for a meal

Kishk: a breakfast cereal to serve with thin cream or milk

This traditional ferment has its origins in the Middle East, and it is a perfect combination of complete proteins. The live cultures in the yoghurt will break down the enzyme inhibitors and the phytic acid, and it is one of the very few breakfast cereals that is truly a healthy food. Kishk has many variations, but as a breakfast cereal it could have a very important role to play for all family members. Try different grains but make sure the berries are cracked into several pieces before adding the yoghurt to ferment.

4 cups cracked wheat or bulgur   4 cups yoghurt

1. Mix the ingredients in a bowl, cover with a tea towel and allow to ferment for 24 hours in a dark place
2. Spread the mixture as thin as possible on an oiled biscuit tray and dry out at a temperature up to 65°C in the oven or in a dehydrator
3. When the mixture has dried, place it in batches in the food processor and pulse lightly until coarsely crumbled. Store in airtight containers in the fridge

You can add more interest to the plain kishk by adding dried fruit, activated nuts, desiccated coconut and some coconut sugar for sweetening. Use it as a breakfast cereal.

Soured Porridge Pot

1. Place 2-3 cups of oats in a bowl or large jar with enough water so that it swims a bit

2. Add a couple of tablespoons of sour whey, kefir, buttermilk or yoghurt to introduce some lactic forming bacteria into the mix

3. Let it sit in a warm place for a few days or until it starts to smell sour and have little bubbles

4. Every time you take out the fermented slurry to cook into porridge, make sure to leave about one cup in the jar and add some more oats and water to the mixture

5. Leave for around 48 hours to ferment

6. When cooking the porridge, add enough water in the pot to cover by 2 centimetres then cook into a porridge until it has thickened

Five Grain Cereal Mix

2 cups wheat or spelt berries

2 cups barley or oats

2 cups millet

2 cup split peas or lentils

2 cups short grain rice

This combination conforms to the Yellow Emperor's classic of internal medicine.

Grind the grains coarsely through a flour mill or thermomix and mix together.

Five Grain Fermented Porridge

1. Add one cup of water to one cup of the cereal mix with half a teaspoon salt, 2 tablespoons sour whey, buttermilk or yoghurt, and stand at room temperature for 24 hours

2. Bring a cup of water to the boil and add the fermented cereal mixture to the pan and bring back to the boil and simmer for several minutes

Serve with cultured butter or sour cream and some coconut sugar or any other natural sweetener.

Ama Koji (a rice ferment)

The starter culture can be bought through GEM cultures among many other outlets online.

A koji is mostly a rice-based ferment of mould-based organisms that will break the complex starches of the rice grains into simpler sugars. The rice itself will be covered by the mycelium overgrowth turning the rice grains into a solid cake. A koji must be bought or made before you can ferment this thin rice porridge. The resulting fermented rice porridge will turn into ama koji and can become much more than a porridge as there are other uses for it too.

The ama koji can be used as a seasoning, marinade, making pickles, and as a sweet treat. As a marinade, ama koji will turn tough meat into a tender cut, cheap fish can be turned into delectable morsels, and any vegetable can be buried within the porridge overnight and softened, sweetened and made more nutritious by the fermenting process. Fermented food browns very quickly in the frying pan so be prepared for a much shorter cooking time. Another way to use ama kjoi is as a sweet dessert served cold with fruit. If you leave the pieces of fruit to ferment in the ama koji overnight, this will change the texture and the flavour of the fruit to a naturally sweetened treat.

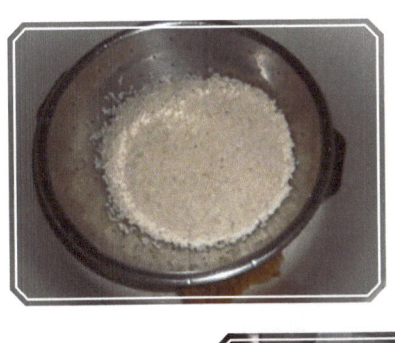 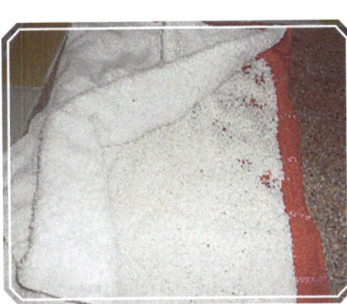 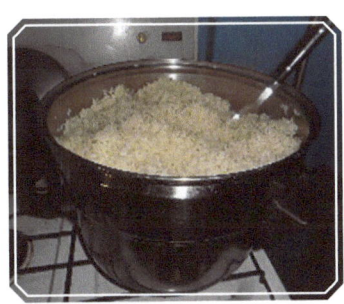

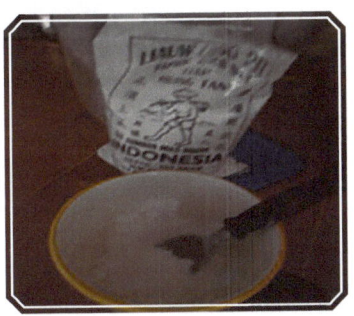 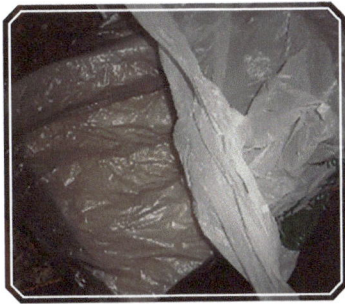

How to make the koji

Koji

1 kilo of medium grain white rice

A steamer

Tray that will fit inside the incubator

2 towels

Baking paper

Thermometer

Soak the rice overnight, drain in a colander, then dry between two towels on a tray, steam the rice for 20 minutes or until just tender.

1. Cool rice to below 50°C, add the starter culture into ¼ of a cup of tapioca starch or flour, mix thoroughly and add to the rice, stirring thoroughly to incorporate all the mould starter around each grain of rice

2. Line a metal tray with kitchen paper and pour the rice mixture into the tray. Fold the remainder of the kitchen paper over the top of the rice then wrap a plastic shopping bag over the tray

3. Place in an incubator for around 40 hours at 30°C. When the fermentation is complete the rice will smell sweet and become caked together into one solid mass

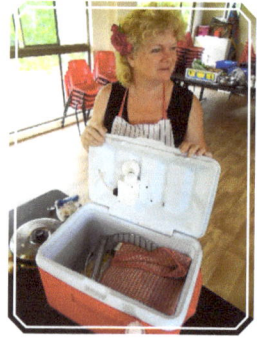 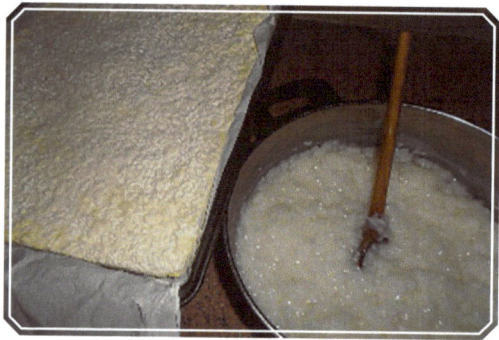 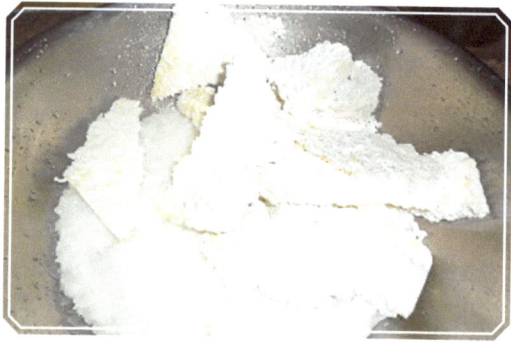

Homemade incubator made with a cool box and a dimmer switch installed in the lid with an incandescent light bulb for warmth. The bulb used in this box is 40 watt. You can also use a reptile warming mat in a coolite box.

The koji can be used immediately or stored in the fridge for about a month or in the freezer for up to 6 months. Koji can also be dried if it is spread out in a very thin layer in a tray and dried until it becomes crisp. It will store and remain viable for up to 6 months. Frozen, the dried koji will keep up to a year if protected from freezer burn

Thin porridge to make Ama Koji

1 cup of short grain white rice   9 cups of water

1. Place the rice and water in a pan. Bring the water to the boil and cook over medium heat for about 20-30 minutes, stirring intermittently until the rice is totally cooked. Cool to around 50–60°C

2. Break up the koji into fine pieces, add to the thin porridge and mix thoroughly

3. Place the entire mixture into a 5-cup rice cooker and use the 'keep warm' function to keep the temperature between 50 and 60°C. Leave to sit for 6 to 10 hours while stirring intermittently to keep the heat evenly distributed

The fermented rice porridge is now turned into ama koiji and is ready to eat, marinade or pickle food with. It is a very gentle sweetness and very easy to digest.

You can store ama koji in the fridge for up to one week; otherwise freeze it in small containers until ready to use.

Amazaki

I like to add one cup of water to one cup of ama koji and let it sit on the bench for a couple of days. The sweetness will be fermented out to become a slightly lactic drink and it's a delicious and refreshing drink with a little bit of grated ginger added. Leave to sit for longer at room temperature and the solids will separate out and you will have the equivalent of sour whey to use for other ferments.

Fermented Brown Rice

Brown rice is high in phytic acid and soaking in water will not effectively eliminate it because brown rice lacks the enzyme phytase. Phytase releases phosphorus and this can be activated by fermentation. The soaking water will need the addition of sour whey added to it so that the phosphorus will become available.

Prepare the brown rice before cooking

cups brown rice

tablespoons sour whey/ water kefir

6½ cups water

1. Place rice, whey and water in a bowl and leave for at least 7 hours or overnight

2. Drain all soaking water into a jar and place in the fridge as this will become the soaking water for the next time

3. Rinse the soaked rice with fresh water and add 2½ cups water into the rice cooker with the fermented rice. Turn on the rice cooker and keep the lid on and cook for about 45 minutes or until cooked

4. Stir in 1 teaspoon sea salt and 2 to 4 tablespoons butter towards the end stage of cooking

NB: Next time you cook brown rice add another few tablespoons of sour whey to the soaking water. After this you won't need to add anymore as the lactic bacteria will have built up enough to keep going by themselves. Always save the soaking water as subsequent batches of brown rice will become softer and fluffier and more digestible. For the next batch, top up with some water as required as the rice must always be covered for the fermenting period. The water can be kept for many years in a jar in the fridge in between soaking the rice on the bench.

Fermented Legumes

Wise wisdom of the past told of soaking and fermenting all legumes before cooking them. As with grains, nuts and seeds, legumes also have inhibitors for nutrient uptake. Lectins and anti-nutrients such as enzyme inhibitors and phytates are the culprits, and soaking legumes in water with some sour whey for 12 to 24 hours is sufficient to neutralise most of them. Soaking also leaches out tannins and indigestible saccharides.

Undercooked beans are not good for you and cooking legumes in a slow cooker is also not a good practice due to the lectins (proteins) not being broken down enough. The cooking water must reach boiling temperature and stay there for at least ten minutes for this reason. Lectins can harm the lining of the intestines, especially the microvilli. This happens when the lectins bind to the protein receptors in the intestinal lining, causing damage.

When the intestines are damaged, lectins, and the foods that they bind to, can pass through the intestinal wall and into the blood stream. These sticky proteins can then wreak havoc in the bloodstream. Once lectins are floating around in the bloodstream, they can bind to any carbohydrate containing protein cells, including insulin and leptin receptors and desensitise them. (More research is needed for this.)

Without proper insulin and leptin function, problems like diabetes and metabolic syndrome can emerge. Lectins may cause insulin and leptin resistance, two major factors in obesity and diabetes. For many, avoiding lectins, especially for a year or so, can help heal the intestinal lining, promote weight loss, reduce allergy symptoms and improve health.

This is the reason why we don't eat raw grains and legumes. Lectins as well as the other nasties need to be fermented out and the legumes cooked until they are soft.

Soy is the most contentious of all the legume family. The soybean has been hailed as a super food providing cheap protein for a growing world population. When you look at the minerals contained in soy products, the manufacturers would have you believe that you are getting a lot of nutrients for your money, but little of the magnesium, calcium, zinc or iron will be assimilated as soy is the worst culprit of all the legume family, with phytic acid and enzyme inhibitors. These play havoc with our digestion. Soymilk, tofu and other soy products that are processed in the factory will leave you mineral-poor and unless you consume traditionally fermented soy it would be better to avoid this legume altogether.

Fermented soybeans on the other hand generate a great number of vitamins and amino acids (proteins) and increased nutrients such as kalium, magnesium and fibre. Miso is full of saponins, lecithin as well as isoflavones, an estrogen-like effect that influences our hormone levels. It can have great benefits for menopausal women but thinking that soy is a cheap way to provide protein for the masses is not wise. Soy needs to be totally broken down to become the super food it is claimed to be and only the traditional soy fermented foods such as miso, soy sauce, natto and tempeh should be consumed. Soy should not be eaten in large quantities due to the hormonal effect on the human endocrine system.

What is not so speculative is that once you are leptin-resistant, you become obese and insulin resistant, and at that point you are intolerant to any type of carbohydrate. This may explain why carbohydrate restriction works in weight loss and improves health.

Cooked and prepared legumes can also be fermented. If you have some bought hummus you can value add to it with fermentation. Stir in a tablespoon of sour whey/ water kefir and stand at room temperature for 24 to 48 hours before placing it in the fridge.

Miso

Miso has an anti-mutagenic effect against mutagenic substances such as tobacco smoke, exhaust gas and scorched meat. When frying or barbequing meat, adding some raw miso to the meal will help to counteract the carcinogenic effect of the burnt meat. Burnt meat has amines all through it and they are carcinogenic. Cutting the burnt part off won't help as these amines have formed right throughout the meat. Barbequing is not such a good idea unless the meat is cooked gently without burning any of it. Miso can also help to eliminate radioactive substances, and it has the effect of rejuvenating damaged cells. Apparently, miso was generously handed out in the aftermath of the bombing of Hiroshima to help counteract the damaging effects of radiation.

Linoleic acid is also found in miso, and this is good for the complexion. There is also a claim that it prevents aging as the free radicals that come about with the oxidation of lipids destroy cell function, and the miso, which is high in vitamin E and therefore rich in antioxidants, will help to halt this destructive process.

The brown colour in miso is called malanoidine and this is the substance that has the suppressive action over the production of fat peroxide.

Miso also scavenges free radicals which become carcinogenic.

To make miso, a koji is needed before the soybeans can break down. A koji is a substrate of mould spores grown on a base of rice or barley, although the Korean method of making miso uses the soybeans to grow the miso mould spores on. The mould spores, aspergillus oryzae, can be purchased through GEM cultures and many other outlets found online anywhere in the world. For this modern style koji you will need a controlled environment to incubate the mould onto the rice at 30°C. You can find the recipe for modern koji in the ama koji recipe in this book

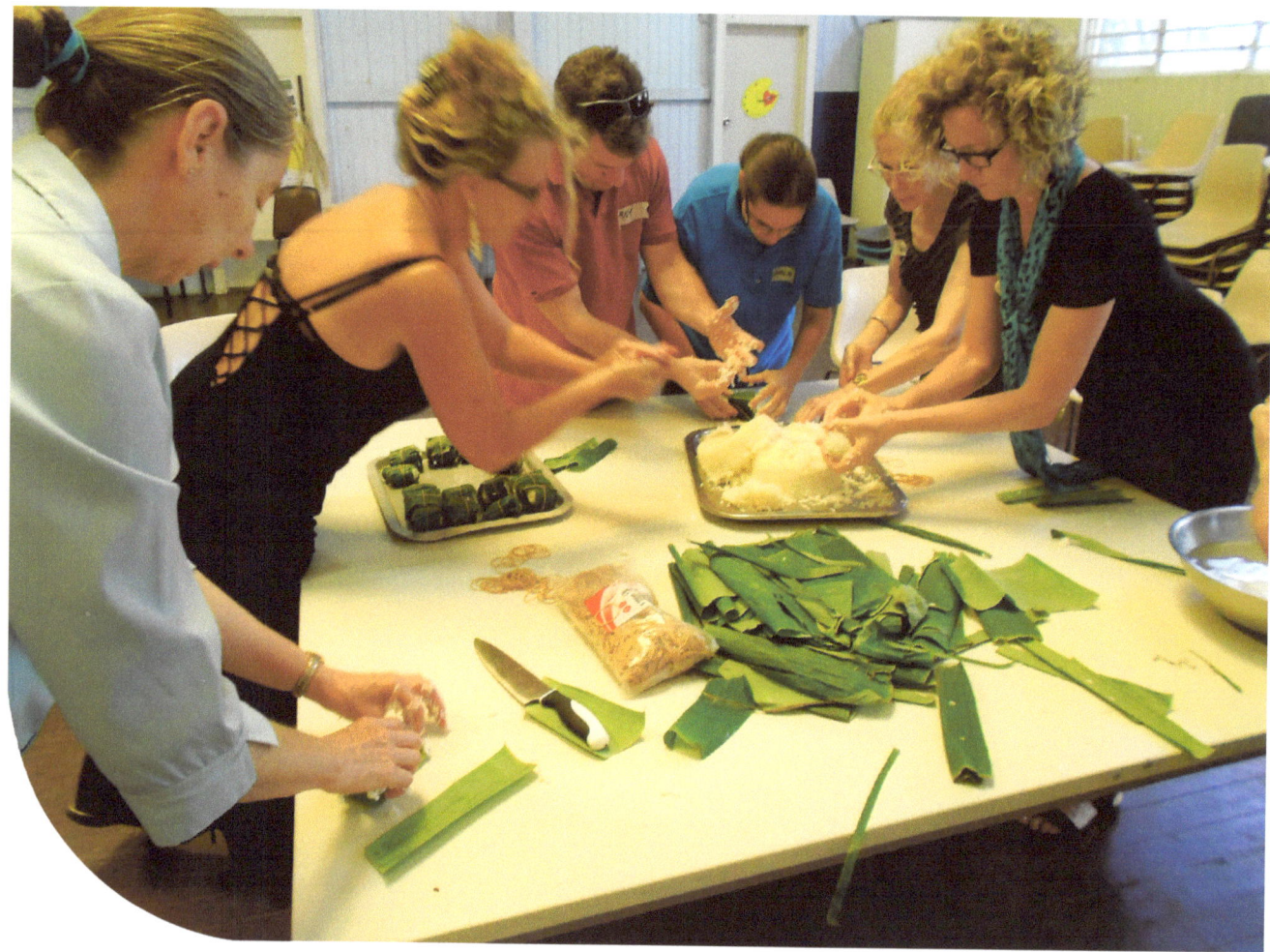

How to make old-fashioned koji

Five cups of rice to five cups of water

1. Steam or boil some medium grain white rice. Make sure the rice is quite dry and sticky when cooked. A rice cooker with one cup of rice to one cup of water makes for a perfect consistency

2. Allow to cool

3. Take handfuls of the rice and roll into balls of about 6 cm in diameter

4. Take strips of banana leaves and wrap them around the balls. The banana leaves have the right kind of spores to make miso with and will inoculate the rice balls over a period of several weeks

5. Wrap elastic bands around the balls to keep the banana strips in place and store them on a rack for maximum airflow

6. Cover with a lace tablecloth or curtain so birds and vermin can't get to the koji balls

They should be kept out of the weather and direct sunshine. The balls should be ready for use in about one to two months. The colours should be yellow, green and black. Orange and red colours are not from the right kind of moulds and these balls should be discarded. The moisture in the air may have been too damp to allow the rice to dry out enough in time. Koji is traditionally made in the cooler time of the year, and the atmosphere should not be too dry as the moulds won't have a chance to grow on the rice balls before they dry out completely.

When the koji balls are ready, unwrap the dried banana leaves and store them in an airtight container until they are needed. When you are ready to make miso, rinse the koji balls, add a sprinkle of water over it and allow them to soften overnight to rehydrate the rice before adding to the cooked soybeans the following day.

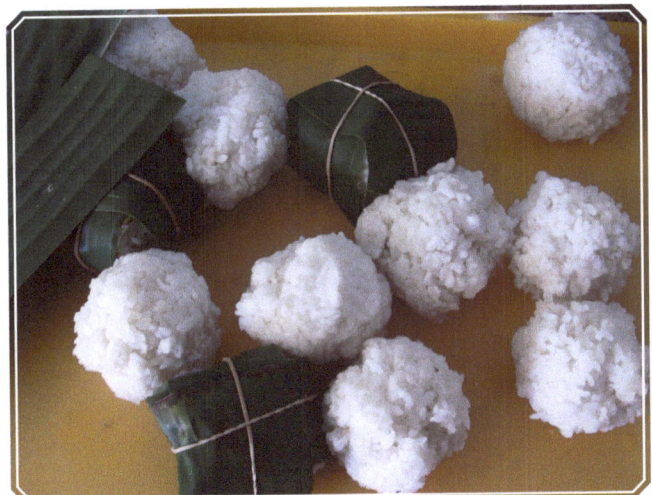
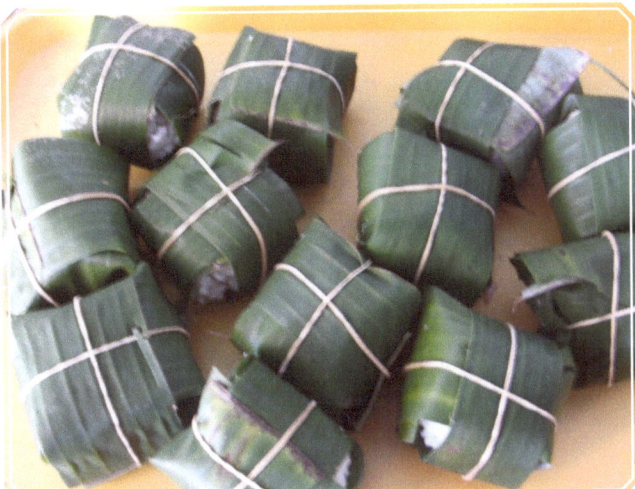

Making the Miso

Instead of using koji balls for making miso you can use the modern koji method as described in making ama koji. Follow the recipe but omit the thin porridge. Both the koji balls and the pure cultures have a viable life for up to six months in the fridge. After this time there is no guarantee that the koji will be active enough to make miso successfully.

There are three basic koji types for miso:

Rice miso → Barley miso → Soybean miso

These are made into sweet, mild and salty miso. There are many different miso styles and below are three to choose from. Shiro, white or sweet, miso is a fast miso, Edo miso is a mid-term ferment, and Hatcho miso is a dark and salty miso. All mature and improve with age.

Shiro miso

500 grams dry soybeans

1kilo koji

125 grams coarse sea salt

fermenting time 3–5 weeks

Edo miso

400 grams dry soybeans

500 grams dry koji

200 grams coarse sea salt

fermenting time 6–12 months, 18 months is even better

Hatcho miso

1750 grams dry soybeans

1250 grams dry koji

750 grams coarse sea salt

fermenting time 18 months

Select the style miso you wish to make and measure the dry amounts of soybeans, koji and salt. (You also need to determine if you are going to use koji balls or a modern koji)

1. Soak the soybeans overnight in plenty of water with the addition of some sour whey/ water kefir

2. The following day, drain and add plenty of fresh water and cook until the beans are soft enough to squash between your little finger and thumb

3. You can whiz the soybeans, salt and koji in a food processor but the traditional method is to aim for a slightly textured miso. You can achieve this by placing some of the mix into a plastic bag and using a rolling pin to mash the beans and not turning it into a fine paste but keeping it slightly textured. The miso mix should be of ear lobe consistency so have a feel of your ear lobe before getting your hands into the miso mix. You can add some of the leftover soy cooking water to add to the mix if it is too dry

4. Add most of the salt to the soybean mix and scatter some of the leftover salt into the bottom of a clean container such as a small crock or a food grade plastic container

5. Add a tablespoon of miso from a previous batch to seed it with the right microbes and mix thoroughly

6. Throw in small handfuls of miso to force the air out while packing the jar and try to have a good aim to avoid making a mess

7. Even out the miso mix with your hand in the pot. Scatter the leftover salt on top and place some grease-proof paper over it

8. Cover with plastic wrap and label the container with the starting and finishing date and the style miso. Any liquid that forms on top of your miso is tamari and should be left until the miso is matured

9. The miso will need to be checked every couple of months for any stray moulds that may be growing on top. Simply scrape off anything that looks foreign. White mould that can grow on top of your miso is harmless and can simply be stirred into the rest of the mixture or scraped off

Leave the miso in an even temperature and a dark place.
Try to leave it as long as you can, as the longer it is kept, the better it becomes.
The best kind of miso is at least two years old.

Tempeh

You will need a large saucepan, a large bowl, stirring spoon, tray, 2 hand towels, clip lock plastic sandwich bags, tempeh mould, a thermometer and an incubator set at 30°C

Rhizophus oligosporus
(You can source tempeh starter from topcultures.com)

Making the Tempeh

3 cups/ 600 grams soybeans, washed and drained	6 cups water

1. Bring the soybeans to the boil, turn off the heat and leave overnight; or bring the soybeans to the boil and cook for 20 minutes then leave for 2 hours

2. Rub the soybeans vigorously between the hands to loosen the hulls and split the beans. Pour plenty of water into the pot, stir the beans around and leave the beans to sink for a few seconds. Pour off the hulls floating on the top. Do this several times until most of the hulls are poured off

3. Add enough water to cover the soybeans with a dash of vinegar and allow the beans to boil on medium heat for 40 minutes

4. Drain

5. Have a tray ready with two hand towels. Line the tray with a hand towel and pour the soybeans onto the tray. Place the other hand towel on top and rub the beans around to soak up as much excess moisture as possible

6. Spread the cooked soybeans on a tray and leave them in the sun or a slow oven to dry out as much as possible, as moisture will prevent the mould growing properly over the soybeans

7. Place the beans in a large mixing bowl

8. Add 1 teaspoon of the tempeh mould mixed in a ¼ cup of tapioca starch or flour and stir thoroughly into the soybeans

9. Take 3 clip lock sandwich bags and punch holes at ½ inch/ 1 cm intervals. You can use the pointy end of the scissors or a thick needle with a couple of hand towels underneath, or I use a leather awl that does the job beautifully

10. Fill the bags evenly and neaten them, as whatever shape the beans are in the bag is how they will look when the mould spores have brought all the soybeans together into a solid cake

11. Place the filled bags in the incubator on a metal wire tray to ensure good air circulation and set the temperature just below 30°C keeping the bags as far away from the heat source as possible. Placing a tea towel over the packets will also prevent overheating from any light source

12. Check the temperature at regular intervals as the beans will heat up after twelve hours. Aim to get the temperature just under 30°C. If the temperature reaches over 35°C it will kill the mould spores and the tempeh making process won't be successful

After 12 to 24 hours, you should notice a dulling appearance over the soybeans and when the tempeh ferment is complete after about 30 hours you will see a beautiful even covering of white mould over the soybeans. When the whole packet is covered with a solid mass of white mould spores, you can place the bags in the fridge or freezer. Make sure that the tempeh packets are separated from each other in the fridge as they keep generating heat.

After they have been in the fridge for a week, you may notice some black spots appearing over the tempeh. This is a sign of the mould maturing and it is sporulating or able to reproduce itself. If you would like to recapture the mould spores then allow the tempeh to become quite black in places and slice very thinly and place on a fine wire mesh tray to dry until the pieces are crisp and crunchy. Place the dried tempeh pieces in the food processor and whiz until you see the dust of the mould in the container. Pour the whole lot into a sieve and you will find that the mould spores will come through and the soybeans will be separated out and left inside the sieve. Keep it in a jar in the fridge and date it as it will be viable for up to six months. Use as directed in the instructions.

Fermented Bean Pate

This ferment is great for using in tacos as a refried bean mix. I love spreading it on my sourdough wraps

I can of soft beans such as butter or cannellini

1 can of borlotti or pinto beans

½ an onion

2 garlic cloves, crushed and peeled

Small knob of ginger

sea salt to taste

chili or spice blend to taste (I love barbeque charcoal seasoning)

2 tablespoons sour whey/ water kefir

1. Add the drained butter/ cannelini beans and process until smooth with the ingredients except for the borlotti/ pinto beans

2. Place the bean mix into a bowl and add the drained borlotti beans and mix well

3. Bottle into glass jars making sure to leave at least 2-3 cm for expansion. If there isn't enough room for the bean mix to rise. it will blow the lid off the jar.

4. Leave at room temperature for about 2 days or when signs of fermentation are seen

You can use any other spices to jazz up the fermented bean paste including hot chillies, cumin and all spice.

Trust your instincts and not your preconceived ideas of food that may have gone off when they ferment. On the contrary, the fermented legumes are made much more digestible and pleasant to eat.

NB: A variation to this ferment is to add some water kefir or sour whey to a tub of hommus and ferment for 24 – 48 hours on the bench. Any purchased bean-based dip can be turned into a ferment for enhanced flavour and digestibility.

Fermented Vegetables and Fruits

Any vegetable can be fermented and, depending on their firmness, most will do well by immersing them in water. Some examples of fermented vegetables are sauerkraut, kimchi and pickled cucumbers. These are examples of lactic ferments, and they contribute to good digestion at any meal. Fermented vegetables tend to be much more pronounced in flavour and only a small quantity needs to be eaten at any one time for their benefits. They also make a great substitute for a garden salad as sometimes there simply aren't any greens in the garden. A great advantage of fermenting your vegetables and fruit is that the pesticide residues of chemically grown produce are largely fermented out, so their toxic effects won't have a detrimental effect on your health. It is always better though to have organically grown food so that you have more nutrients, as hybrid plants aren't as nutritious as open pollinated plants.

Fruit can also be fermented. It is advisable to start with dried fruit as these are more stable to ferment with. There are a lot of sugars in fruit, and these can easily turn to alcohol instead of turning slightly lactic and maintaining their sweetness. Fermenting with fruit, especially fresh fruit, will need closer monitoring than with other foods but they can be turned into a myriad of delicious pastes and spreads.

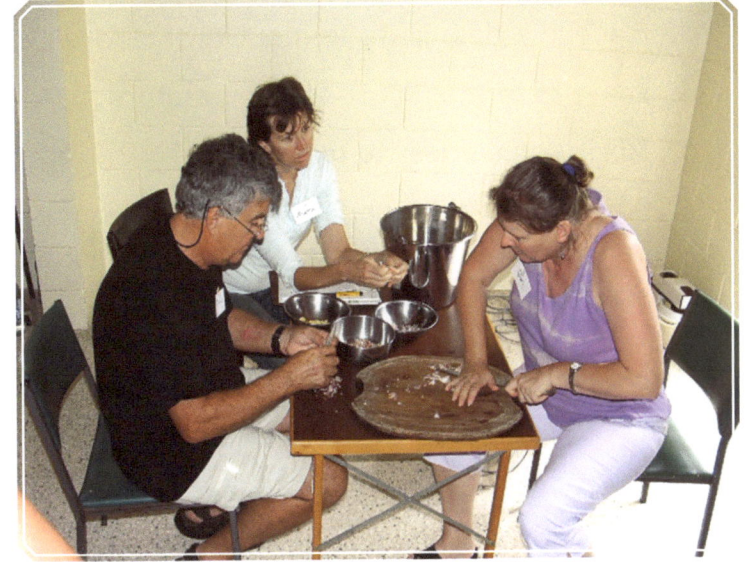

Fermented Apricot Spread

This is a great substitute for jam on your morning toast. There is no need for highly sugared jams on bread when you can enjoy this tasty fruit ferment. Feel free to try other dried and fresh fruits.

4 cups fresh apricots or the equivalent of dried apricots soaked in water overnight

I teaspoon sea salt

2 tablespoons sour whey/ water kefir

1 stick cinnamon

1 star anise

2 cloves

Honey to taste

1. If you are using fresh apricots, peel off skin and remove the pip. Puree in a food processor until smooth. If you are using dried apricots, cover with warm water and let them rehydrate overnight. Once softened, puree until smooth

2. Mix in the salt and the whole spices

3. Place in a glass jar to ferment

4. Leave to ferment at room temperature for 12–24 hours

5. Mix in some honey to taste

6. Store in the fridge and it should last about a month. If you have more than required, it can be frozen in containers as the fermentation does not stop in the fridge, but it does slow it right down

Use this apricot spread in place of jam and it's also good on roast pork.

Fermented Raisin Chutney

Raisins add their sweetness in this ferment, and with the addition of spices will pleasantly surprise you with its sweet and pungent savoury flavours

1 cup raisins, soaked in water for at least an hour

1 clove of garlic, peeled and crushed

¼ cup finely minced coriander leaves

10 black peppercorns

1/4 teaspoon red chili flakes or powder

1 tablespoon ground coriander seeds and 1/2 tablespoon cumin seeds

1 teaspoon freshly grated ginger

½ teaspoon sea salt

1 tablespoon sour whey/water kefir

approx. ½ cup water

1. Whiz the raisins along with the soaking water into the food processer with the peppercorns, chilli flakes/powder, garlic and ginger

2. Pulse the processor a few times until the mixture is a chunky paste

3. Add the coriander and cumin seeds after pounding them with a mortar and pestle (you can blitz them too)

4. Add the chopped fresh coriander

5. Transfer the chutney into a clean glass jar

6. Mix the salt into the water with the whey/ water kefir, then pour it into the jar to cover the fruit. Cover the top with a clip lock sealed bag with a little water in it to keep the raisins from bobbing up above the water line, and close the lid Set the jar on the counter for two to three days. Taste to see when it is lactic enough, then place in the fridge where it will store for a couple of weeks

This chutney is a great accompaniment to meats and curries

Fermented Pineapple/ Mango Chutney

This is another version of the fermented fruit spread. Keep an eye on the consistency otherwise it will ferment down into mush if it is too liquid.

3 cups of chopped pineapple or mango

½ small minced red onion

½ chopped orange or red capsicum

½ cup chopped fresh coriander

1½ teaspoons sea salt

2 tablespoons sour whey/ water kefir

¼ cup lime or lemon juice

1 tablespoon grated ginger

½ teas red chili pepper, fresh or dried

½ cup water (as needed to keep the contents submerged)

1. Mix all the ingredients together except for the water and pour into a large glass jar

2. Add the water and make sure all the ingredients are below the water line with enough room for the chutney to expand

3. Ferment for 12 hours then store in the fridge. Make sure all the ingredients are kept under the water line to stop them from growing white mould on top. If there are some white bits floating on top, then lift these off.

Fermented Fruit Paste

Quite a few years ago I was introduced to a fruit kimchi by a fermenting friend. It was a very colourful assembly of different kinds of fruits such as apples, rock melon, pineapple, and there were also root vegetables such as parsnips and carrots. When I was asked to try some, I was not impressed. I found the parsnips were overtaking the flavour of the fruits and I decided to vary the recipe. I left out all the vegetables and added dried fruit to the fresh fruit. Eventually dates became the base and some prunes were added for moisture and texture. It has become a fermented fruit paste and who knows, this recipe may change by this time next year!

This is a lactic ferment that will serve as a dessert, or as a snack whenever you are feeling peckish. Dates are the basis of this recipe, and the amount used should exceed the rest as they are the secret to giving that lovely fudgy flavour and natural sweetness. This lactic ferment doesn't taste sour due to those date sugars. The amounts are approximate.

750 grams of pitted dates, cut in half

250 grams pitted prunes cut in half

150 grams of a combination of soft nuts and seeds. Larger nuts such as cashews, walnuts, pecans etc. should be coarsely cut.

100 grams of finely cut up pineapple, rock melon, apple or any other firm fruit

A bit of grated ginger

1. Have a four-litre bucket ready and fill with approximately ½ litre of water

2. Add enough salt in the water to be able to taste a slight saltiness and add some soured whey/ water kefir to inoculate the new batch with lactic forming bacteria

3. After mixing all the dry ingredients together, add to the prepared liquid in the bucket and place another bucket of the same size inside to press down onto the fruit mix. Just a little water needs to cover the ingredients so that everything is submerged underneath the liquid. Any surplus water that can't be absorbed by the dates will be lost and that will include all those lovely date sugars

4. Weigh the inside bucket down with a large glass jar filled with water. Allow the ferment to stand at room temperature for five days and then transfer the ingredients into a glass jar. There should be virtually no liquid left after the dates have absorbed it all. If too much water is added to the mixture, then it will become alcoholic.

Your fermented fruit paste is now ready to eat. It's great to serve with kefir milk or yoghurt with a dollop of soured cream. This ferment will keep for a very long time in the fridge although it might not last that long when people catch on how good it is. This fermented fruit paste recipe can also be used as the filling for fruit mince tarts or turned into probiotic rum balls by blitzing the fruit paste to a fine consistency with the addition of a little rum and enough cocoa powder to make the mixture firm enough. Roll the mixture into small balls and roll them into desiccated coconut.

Sauerkraut

Sauerkraut is made from cabbage and any of the solid heading varieties can be used. The red cabbage is fun to work with as the colour is so vibrant. Used on its own it makes a very red sauerkraut, but when it is mixed with the green cabbage, the colour becomes pink and then to a light greenish up the top of the jar. My preferred cabbage is sugarloaf as the sauerkraut takes only a week or two before it is soft and moreish to eat. The other cabbage varieties will take several weeks before they are ready to eat but they will keep a very long time in the fridge whereas the sugarloaf will turn to mush after about six week. There is no need to add anything to the sauerkraut-making process except a little salt. The lactic forming bacteria are already present on the cabbage itself. As a rule, if you want your sauerkraut to stay crisp and crunchy, add more salt; if you would like your sauerkraut to go soft and mild, use less salt.

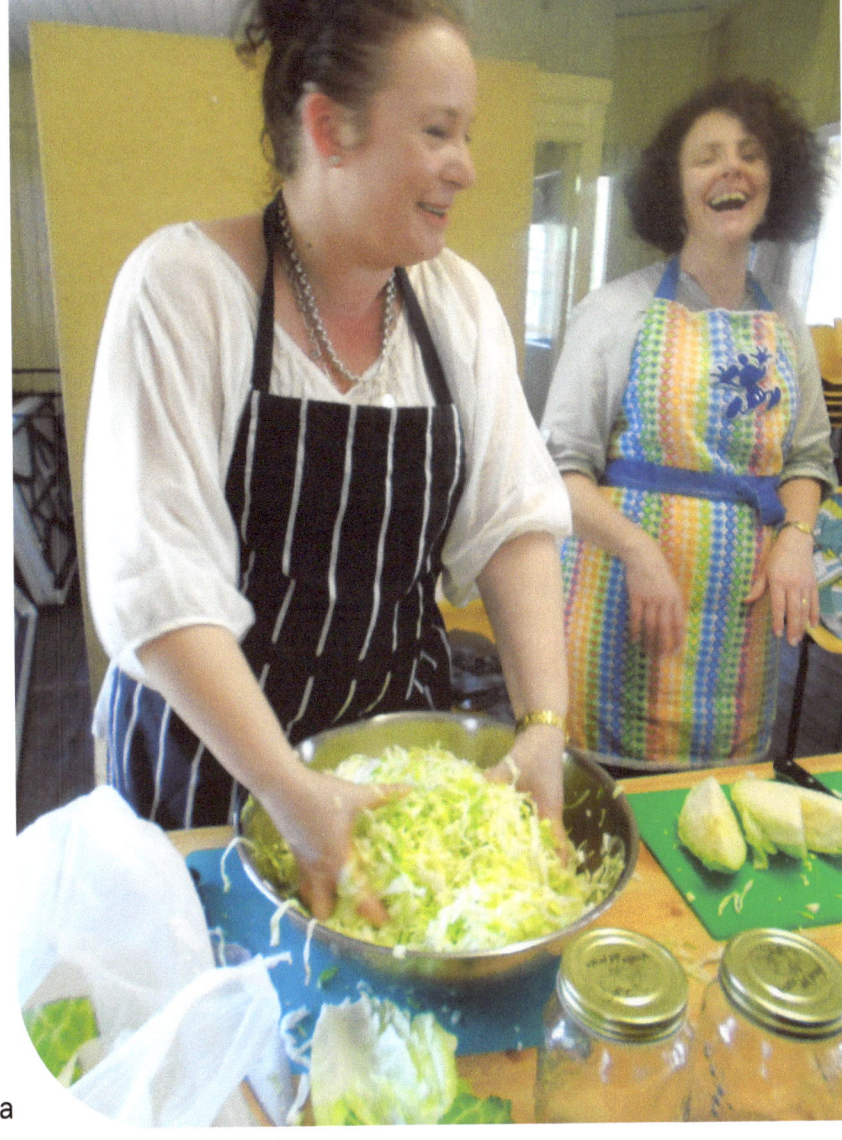

Take the green outer leaves from the cabbage and put them aside for later.

1. Shred the cabbage very fine – a mandolin can be useful
2. Place it all in a large bowl and work with your hands to release the juices You will need to work hard to draw out all the cabbage juices to the point where you can squeeze it and lots of juice comes dripping out

3. Sprinkle a couple of pinches of salt to help draw out the juices. You can also add some caraway seed for taste or any other spices such as juniper berries

4. Pack tightly into a wide-mouthed glass jar

5. Keep the cabbage submerged by placing some scrunched up outer cabbage leaves into the jar to keep the cabbage submerged under its own liquid. The leaves may get a bit mouldy after 5 days, but this won't affect the quality of the sauerkraut

6. Let it stand at room temperature for a couple of weeks or so and pour off any excess sauerkraut juice and bottle it for a wonderful pick-me-up tonic. Push the sauerkraut down hard into the jar so that there are no air pockets and try to have a little of the juice sit on top

7. Keep the sauerkraut in the fridge after a few weeks on the bench, and if there is some mould growing on top, scrape it off, as underneath it will be quite healthy

It's important to check the sauerkraut once a week so it doesn't spoil but in very hot weather, I will keep it in the fridge to mature after two weeks on the bench.

Kimchi

Take a wongbok cabbage and cut it in half lengthwise and then halve again lengthwise, then chop into pieces with four or five cuts along the length of the wongbok to make large coarse pieces. Place in a large bowl and bash the cut wongbok with the end of a rolling pin or a kraut pounder. This will help to break down the cellulose fibres prior to fermentation.

2 tablespoons sour whey/ water kefir/ sauerkraut juice

½ to ¾ litres water

3–4 red hot chillies, finely chopped (alternatively you can buy Korean chili powder at an Asian supermarket – use 1 dessertspoon per wongbok cabbage)

1 teaspoon of sea salt

Optional: add 1–2 onions, leeks or scallions, thinly sliced, 1–2 carrots, thinly sliced and some fresh grated ginger

1. Mix a brine of about ½ to ¾ litre of water in a fermenting bucket or container for one wongbok cabbage and add a teaspoon of salt, testing to see if the water tastes slightly salty then add some sour whey and the chili spices

2. I also like to add a dessertspoon of paprika powder to add to the red colour. Add any other ingredients into the fermenting bucket. Place a plate on top with a weight on it to keep the vegetables submerged.

3. Keep on a bench for five days then drain off most of the free-running liquid while pressing the fermented wongbok cabbage with your hands. Add some Asian chili paste to the fermented cabbage for a delicious kimchi flavor.

4. Transfer the kimchi into a jar, taking off the surplus liquid while pressing all the cabbage down to exclude any air

5. Save this leftover liquid in a jar and store it in the fridge to use for another batch. The kimchi will be ready to eat in about two to three weeks. Make sure that there is always a bit of liquid sitting on top of the jar to prevent any white mould from forming

Cucumber Kimchi

A few years ago, at the end of summer I had an abundance of cucumbers coming out of the garden and one of the backpackers (wwoofers) that stay here on the farm, a lovely Korean lady by the name of May, gave me this recipe for cucumber kimchi. She stayed here with her friend for several weeks and in that time, we worked our way through a twenty-litre bucket of cucumbers with this delicious kimchi recipe!

I love using the very small cucumbers and leave them whole in the fermenting jar. They last a lot longer without going mushy. Otherwise, Lebanese cucumbers are the best to use for this recipe as they are fleshier than the usual seedy varieties.

1. Take several cucumbers and cut them into fingers

2. Sprinkle with salt and leave for about 20 minutes to draw out the juices Squeeze the cucumber fingers to get rid of the excess juice and salt

3. In a jar or a bucket add some soy sauce, vinegar and a few tablespoons of sour whey/ water kefir to some water. Add chili spices and salt to taste. (There is a Korean chili spice especially for making kimchi that can be bought at Asian supermarkets and gives that authentic taste)

4. Place the cucumber pieces into the jar, add enough water to cover them

5. Leave at room temperature for at least 24 hours before eating. I place a clip lock sandwich bag with water in it to keep the cucumber pieces immersed under the liquid as they may otherwise go mouldy if they are allowed to bob up to the surface

The jar can be kept on the bench for a day to ferment and soften the pickled cucumber pieces but after this, store in the fridge for longer keeping.

Enjoy as a spicy pickle or add to salads.

Carrot kimchi

Salt to taste

2 tablespoons whey/ water kefir

Fish sauce/soy sauce to taste

A dash of vinegar

Julienned carrots

Julienned daikon radish or jicama

Some onion, finely chopped

2 cloves garlic, finely chopped

Some finely grated ginger

Any hot spices to taste

Water

1. Place the julienned root vegetables in a jar and cover with water

2. Add the whey / kefir water and all the spices

3. Keep submerged under the water with a clip lock bag filled with water, a sterilised rock or a glass weight. The water should just cover the vegetables

4. Keep on the bench to ferment until the carrots start to soften, then store in the fridge

This ferment will easily store for up to two months in the fridge and the flavours improve with age. You can eat it when it is to your liking.

Fermented Tomato Sauce

This tomato sauce is a great way to introduce your family to fermented foods. It has just the right blend of spices to make it taste like conventional tomato sauce but with all the benefits of being a probiotic rich food to aid in healthy gut flora. Conventionally grown tomatoes are known for their pesticide residues, but the fermentation will largely negate this by breaking down the toxins. This recipe is simply a guide and is very loose with the number of spices and the other ingredients. The tomato paste helps to give the sauce enough body and a more concentrated tomato flavour and this can also be adjusted according to your own taste. Use vine ripened fresh tomatoes for best results or peeled tomatoes from a tin.

One tin peeled tomato or 3 large fresh tomatoes

1 sachet tomato paste

1 teaspoon Celtic Sea salt/ soy sauce

1 teaspoon smoky paprika

¼ cup maple syrup/ coconut sugar

A few tablespoons of sour whey or water kefir

1. Place all the ingredients into a food processor and blend into a smooth sauce
2. Pour the sauce straight into a used commercial tomato sauce bottle and ferment overnight or 24 hours on the bench

This tomato sauce is a good trick to play on unwitting family members especially if they aren't partial to fermented foods. If you are filling glass bottles or jars, make sure to leave some room for expansion. The sauce lasts for months in the refrigerator, but your family is likely to polish it off much sooner

Nuka Doca

It's been quite a few years since I made some nuka doca. It was fun and it lasted for several months but then it spoiled so I threw it all into the compost bin. I'm not sure if it was the warmer weather of our subtropical climate or because I didn't stir it often enough. Researching for this book has made me interested in making another nuka doca box just for the pure fun of it. I suggest you give this ferment a go and see what you think of it.

The basis for this ferment is roasted rice bran but any other bran will do. The bran is prepared with all sorts of flavours including salt, chili, garlic, ginger – in fact anything that has a pungent flavour.

2 kgs of lightly roasted fresh rice bran

400 grams of unrefined sea salt

2 litres of chemical free water

1 slice of bread

A handful of dried kelp

Sliced chilies

Grated ginger

Nuka doca starter, sour whey or sauerkraut juice

1. A plastic box with a lid to keep the rice bran in is fine and you can keep your nuka doca box in a cool spot in the house. A smaller container such as a crock pot or a glass bowl that will fit in the fridge is advisable in hot weather.

2. Roast the rice bran until it starts to darken into a golden brown.

3. If you can't get hold of some nuka doca starter, sprinkle any other probiotic starter it into the toasted rice bran when it has cooled. This will introduce the lactic bacteria that are needed to start the fermentation process. Add the salt, chilies, kelp and any other flavours such as raw miso.

4. Boil two litres of water, remove from heat and add the torn-up slice of bread. Allow the bread to soften and mash by hand when sufficiently cool. When the water is at room temperature add to the bran mix a little at a time, until you have a dryish mix. Instead of water you can add a litre of kelp broth or even some beer to speed up the fermentation.

You can now see how varied and interesting a nuka doka can be. The moisture content should be at the point where you pick up a handful of the bran mix and squeeze out a few droplets of water.

Lactic bacteria producing colonies that are crucial to the fermentation process, must come from sources such as the skin of the hand and this is done by the daily stirring of the mixture by hand. Adding some fermented vegetables and fruit peelings all help to activate the bran mixture. Keep adding some fruit and vegetable peelings every day and stir thoroughly each time. After about a week the bran will become alive with friendly bacteria and when you smell the lactic ferment in the rice bran your nuka doca is ready to pickle your vegetables.

At this point the starter vegetables and peelings are discarded, and the pickling vegetables are buried in the bed for as little as a few hours to a maximum pickling time of one month. A daily stirring is essential and twice a day in hot weather is important as it keeps the mixture aerated and fresh. If it smells stinky and 'off', you will need to discard it and start again. It is also a good idea to keep adding a bit of lactic fermented vegetables such as sauerkraut over time to keep the mixture alive but the daily stirring by hand is already going to keep adding the friendly bacteria levels needed to keep it fresh. (This should bring the message home that by using antiseptic hand washes we are destroying the friendly bacteria on our skin that are essential to keeping us in good health.) Another tip on keeping the nuka doca fresh is to add some more toasted rice bran and salt once a month when the mixture becomes too moist.

Almost any vegetable can be pickled through the nuka doca, but favourites are mushrooms, eggplant, zucchini, capsicum and cucumber. The taste of the nuka pickles can range from pleasantly tangy to very sour or salty and pungent. These pickles tend to retain their crispness, and they are used as a condiment to the main meals. Meat and fish can also be put through the nuka box. When the pickle is ready for eating, rinse off the rice bran and it is ready for serving. The pickled vegetable should have a gleam and freshness about it and it should taste pungent and rather soft to eat.

Fermented Dairy Products

Raw milk is becoming very popular and while it is illegal to purchase, many people are trying to get hold of it. Cheese made from raw milk tastes so much better and is better for you, as well as butter made from fermented cream. Cultured milk drinks such as kefir and yoghurt are all superior in taste and good health. I have my own cows and goats so I usually have my own supply of raw milk to make my cheese and fermented dairy products, but most people don't have access to raw milk and will have to make do with the pasteurised variety.

When the milk is pasteurised, it undergoes a heating process that is designed to kill any pathogens. The problem is that it kills all the friendly bacteria and enzymes as well and this is where the trouble starts. People who suffer from lactose intolerance will fare better on raw milk as the enzyme lactase will break down the milk sugars when the milk is ingested, but the pasteurising process kills this sugar-digesting enzyme and consequently people can feel bloated and uncomfortable when they drink pasteurised milk.

Lactic-forming bacteria are found in raw milk and these help the milk to sour and turn it into clabbered or curdled milk. Naturally soured milk can be made into quark, and the resulting whey can be used to start new ferments. Milk is also an excellent vehicle to grow many more friendly bacteria that will help with our inner health. Pasteurised milk can be transformed by fermentation and turned back into the healthy living food it was meant to be. Whilst it isn't the same as raw milk with its many diverse strains of bacteria and enzymes, fermenting the milk will make it a much better product. The taste of fermented dairy products is superior, and has many health benefits.

Hygiene is of utmost importance when dealing with milk as it wouldn't do well to grow pathogens whilst growing the beneficial bacteria and enzymes. All utensils need to be hot water rinsed and air-dried (not wiped with a tea towel). The milk used for cheese making should be as fresh as possible to get the best results, except for the making of curdled milk quark with raw milk.

Making cheese

You will need cheese-making cultures to make cheese. Rennet is an enzyme that will set the milk into a solid curd. Use the rennet according to directions as there are various types of rennet available with differing strengths. Cheese-making bacteria are used to influence the texture, and they also help to acidify and mature the cheese. White mould spores can also be purchased to grow the mould on camembert and brie cheese as well as the blue mould for blue vein cheese. I purchase my cheese cultures from Cheeselinks based in Victoria, Australia, but there are many other places you can buy them from. A quick search on the internet from anywhere in the world will get them to you or try various home brew shops in a town near you.

Cheese-making utensils can be improvised from what you can find in your kitchen. A large pot of at least 7 litre capacity is useful and a curd cutting knife can be an icing spatula. A curd cutting knife has a blade that can reach right down to the bottom of the pot. When cutting the cheese curd, the handle of a kitchen knife would otherwise mess up the curd if the blade isn't long enough. To make the horizontal cut you can take the curd knife and cut into the pot at 45-degree angles to make diamond shaped cubes or with a flat round ladle cut just under the surface area of the curd and make horizontal cuts by spiralling down as many times as you can manage till reaching the bottom of the cheese pot. Trays are also very useful for catching the whey from the cheese making, and for the cheddar cheese you will need a cheese press which is easily made by a handy person. Milk to be used for cheese and yoghurt is ideally of the Jersey and Guernsey variety. Their milk is rich with milk solids so it will give you more cheese for your $$ and a thicker set yoghurt. Goat milk for cheese and yoghurt making is best from the Anglo Nubians for the same reasons.

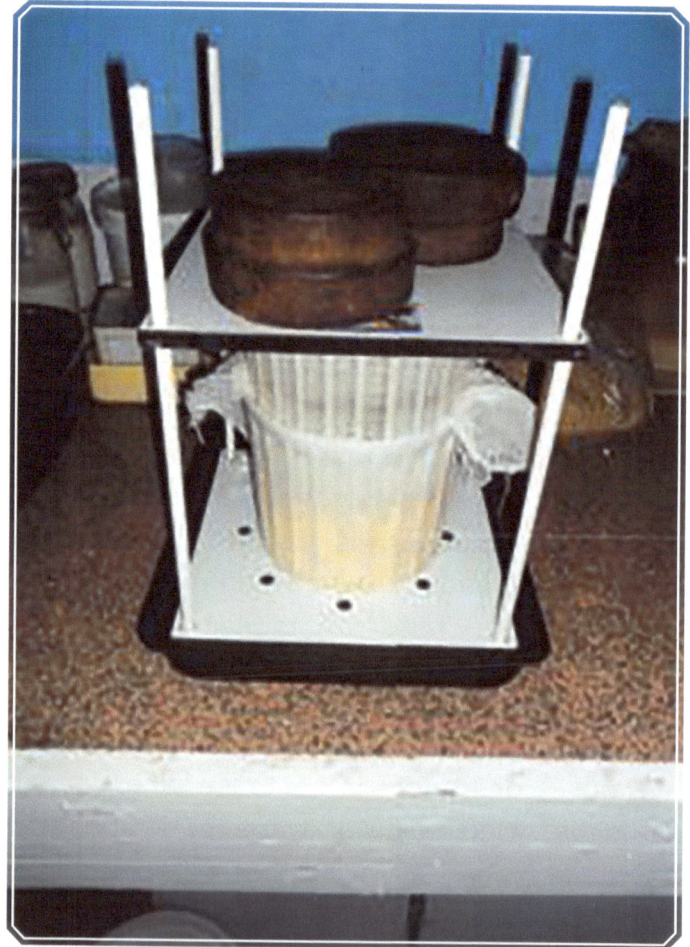

Quark

Making old-fashioned quark is the easiest cheese you'll ever make. This is a spreading cheese, and it is rich in lactic-forming bacteria.

1. Take some raw milk and place it in a glass jar and allow it to curdle at room temperature. If you can't get hold of raw milk, you can use pasteurised milk and add a little pinch of cheese making bacteria to the milk and a little sour whey, yoghurt or kefir water

2. When the milk has thickened and there is some whey visible on the bottom of the jar, the entire contents can be poured into a muslin-lined colander that sits in a large pot or bowl

3. Leave the curds to drain for 24 hours then spoon the curd into a container ready for use

    You can add freshly chopped herbs, salt and pepper and any other flavourings to suit your taste

If the ambient temperature is too cool, find a warm spot to sit the milk in such as an incubator, dehydrator, on top of the fridge or on an electric hot water system. A temperature of around 25–27°C is best.

Don't let it sit any longer than a week.

Make sure everything is very clean.

Neufchattel

A spreading cheese that is sweet and is suitable to spread on bread or crackers.

5 litres of skim or full cream milk

mesophillic cheese starter
bacteria – smidge

rennet – 1 ml (if using chymax)

1. Bring the milk to 20°C and add the starter
2. Add the rennet by diluting it in a tablespoon of water
3. Stir for more than one minute but no more than three
4. Cut the curd after 12 hours with a curd cutting knife in both directions into 1 inch/ two cm spaces and cut diagonally or with spiral cuts to turn into cubes. Leave the curd cubes sit undisturbed in the whey for twelve hours.
5. Ladle the curd into a strainer and allow to drain for 12 hours
6. Add some salt to taste and place into a blender or food processor and whiz until smooth

Add finely chopped garlic chives and grated garlic for a French Boursin type cheese.

Ricotta Cheese

Ricotta cheese is traditionally made either from whole milk, sweet whey, or a combination of both. Although this cheese is not fermented it's included as it uses leftover whey from hard cheese making. Whey should be no more than three hours old after cheese making.

1. Pour the whey into a large pan and add at least 10% whole milk

2. Heat to 95°C

3. Add two tablespoons of vinegar for every litre of fluid, and soon the proteins in the whey will flocculate and rise to the surface. Add more vinegar if nothing much happens at this stage. (Lemon juice will work too)

4. Leave for 5–10 minutes

5. Scoop the curd out of the pan and allow to drain for at least 4–5 hours or overnight in a colander

Butter Kase (A German cheese meaning buttery cheese)

This is a drain curd cheese and it will turn yellow with a rind. It is similar in appearance as a cheddar cheese but much softer and very mild. It is also a washed curd cheese to retard the acidity formation

5 litres cows milk

Thermophillic starter (three grains)

Rennet (2 ml if using chymax rennet)

A round cheese basket with small holes for drainage

1. Bring the milk to 30°C and add the cheese-making bacteria

2. Sit for about 30 minutes to ripen the milk

3. Heat to 40°C, add the rennet, and stir for just under one minute.

4. Cut the curd into half inch / 1 cm cubes

5. Stir the curd very gently at first then more and vigorously over the course of half an hour. Allow the curds to settle for 5 min

6. Pour off 1.3- 1.5 liters of whey to curd level, and add 10% water back into the pot

7. Stir intermittently for ¾ of an hour

8. Ladle the curd into a cheese basket

9. Invert the cheese after several hours and drain for 24 hours

10. Rub about a level dessertspoon of salt on top of the cheese after taking from the cheese basket

11. Leave in the fridge to mature uncovered– approximately 3 weeks. This cheese needs to form a rind so it's best to sit it on a cake cooling rack to allow for maximum airflow. Don't wrap the cheese or it will attract bad moulds. If the cheese becomes covered in grey mould simply wash under the tap with a light scrubbing

Feta

If you would like a very tight-textured feta, use skim milk; a full cream Jersey milk will make a softer textured and very creamy feta. For a cheese basket you will need to look for a straight-sided container and drill lots of small holes on the bottom and on the sides to allow for the drainage of the whey. It is also a good idea to look for a cake cooling rack and sit this over a deep tray to catch the draining whey from the feta cheese. Before turning the cheese curd in the cheese basket after several hours, take the cake cooling rack off the tray, then pour the whey out of the tray and slide the feta upside down still inside the basket onto the tray for the rest of the day until the next day.

6 litres of milk (if using raw milk it helps to use some calcium chloride in addition to ensure the feta stays intact in the brine)

Mesophillic cheese-making bacteria – 1/32nd of a teaspoon (smidge)

Rennet (2 ml if using chymax)

1. Heat the milk to 32–34°C.

2. Add the starter first then the rennet, making sure to stir the rennet for more than one minute but not more than three. Setting time 45 min

3. Cut the curd with a curd cutting knife in both directions into ½ inch or one cm spaces and cut horizontal cuts to have cubes floating in its own whey

4. Rest the curd for five minutes and allow the curd to expel some more of the whey by intermittently stirring for around half an hour. Stir very slowly at first then work your way up to a very vigorous stir in 5-minute increments. Sit the curd in the whey to allow it to settle to the bottom of the pot

5. Ladle the curd into a large strainer sitting in a pot to catch the whey. Leave to drain for half an hour

6. Take the curd down and break up into smaller pieces and ladle into the cheese basket

7. Invert the cheese in its basket several hours later

8. Leave in the basket for another 12 hours then take the cheese out and sprinkle a level dessertspoon of fine salt on top and underneath then place in the fridge on a cake cooling rack

9. Sit the feta on a cake cooling rack until it feels very firm to the touch and not rubbery

10. Longer drying and maturing increases the flavour but generally for 5 days drying in the fridge is good for a mild flavour and firmness. Slice it into neat chunks of about 1 inch/ two cm thick and about eight centimeters long and have a large glass jar ready to place the feta pieces into it and cover with cold water and add some more salt to taste. The feta will stay at least two months in the fridge. I tablespoon of salt for a 6 litre feta is suggested for the brine. The addition of some calcium chloride will keep the feta very firm in the brine

A variation to this feta is to leave it to soak for some time in the whey for a stronger flavor.

Brie Cheese

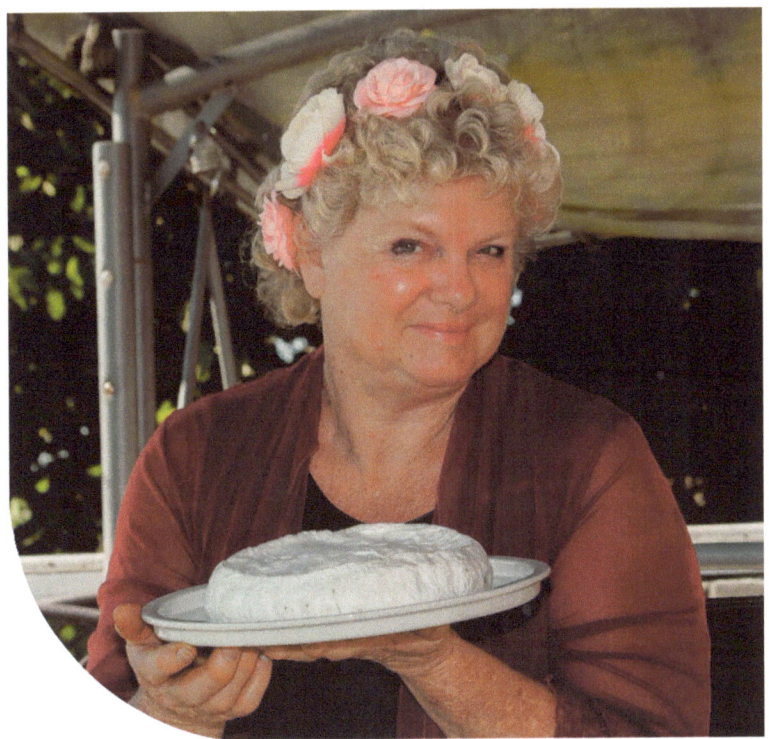

6 litres of cow or goat milk

Mesophilic starter (smidge)

Penicillum candidum
(White mould powder)

Rennet (2 ml if using chymax)

Brie cheese basket and hoop

Cake cooling rack

Tray to catch the whey

1. Heat the milk to 32ºC and add the starter, white mould powder and then the rennet. Stir for more than one minute but no more than three. The milk will set in about 45 min

2. On the bench have the brie cheese basket along with the hoop sitting on a cake cooling rack on the tray and gently ladle the coagulum into it. Cover and leave to drain until it stops dripping

3. Carefully lift the brie basket from the cheese after 36-48 hours. Sprinkle a level dessertspoon of sea salt on top of the cheese and place the Brie on a flat glass plate into the fridge and leave to firm up for several days

4. Place the plate with the Brie in a container with a lid to create a microclimate for the mould to grow on the cheese. Airflow is very important for the microorganisms to thrive so if there is a false bottom in the container the cheese will develop white mould all over. For some fridges this need not be necessary, but most fridges are low in humidity and will not allow the white mould to grow over the cheese

5. Check the brie after a couple of weeks and when you see the mould starting to grow onto the cheese, it can take as long as 4 weeks in a cold fridge and when the brie is fully covered in white mould then you can loosely wrap it in alumium foil to conserve the moisture while ripening the brie

6. It can be eaten at this stage, but it will be very young. Brie is best eaten after 6-8 weeks and can be kept for up to three months but by then the flavour will be very strong, and the cheese is in danger of going off. Take a wedge of the cheese and allow to stand at room temperature in a cheese bell for a few hours to experience the full flavour.

Camembert

4 litres cow/ goat/ sheep milk

Mesophilic starter (smidge)

White mould (penicillum candidum)

Rennet 1.5 ml (if using chymax)

1. Heat the milk to 32ºC and add the starter, penicillum candidum then the rennet. Stir for more than one minute but no more than three

2. Allow the curd to form for about 45 min or until set and cut the curd into 1 inch- 2 cm cubes and leave to sit undisturbed for about 5 minutes

3. Gently heat the curds to 38C.

4. Ladle the curd into small round cheese baskets and place on a wire rack over a tray to catch the whey

5. Allow the whey to drain out for several hours and invert the cheese while keeping it in its basket. The cake cooling rack can be washed and any excess whey should be poured off before inverting the camembert cheeses. Leave until the following day to drain out more whey

6. Sprinkle a level teaspoon of fine salt on top of the cheese and place them in the fridge to firm up. After a few days place them into a microclimate container to encourage the growth of the white mould. Once the camembert is covered in white mould it can be loosely wrapped in aluminum foil or packed into an eco-wrap. This allows the breaking down of fats and proteins in the cheese while conserving moisture. The camembert will feel softer to touch when they are ready to eat

Cheddar Cheese

6 litres of cow milk either raw or pasteurized (not homogenized)

Mesophillic cheese bacteria (smidge)

Rennet 2 ml (if using chymax)

1. Warm the milk to 32°C and add the cheese bacteria

2. Leave to ripen for 20–30 minutes

3. Dilute the rennet into a tablespoon of water in a glass and add to the milk Stir longer than a minute but no more than three

4. When the curd has formed, cut into 1 inch/ 2 cm cubes. Stand for 5 minutes.

5. Slowly heat the curd to raise the temperature to 38°C and make sure to stir the pot as it stops the curd from overheating- this process is called scalding the curd

6. Leave the curd to settle to the bottom for 30 minutes- this is pitching the curd

7. Place the curd into a strainer to drain for an hour

8. Cut the curd into large chunks, lay the curd pieces over each other, repeat again in 15 minutes- this is the cheddaring process to drain off more whey

9. Take the curd and break into walnut sized pieces- this is milling the curd

10. Add one tablespoon of fine sea salt

11. Prepare the cloth to fit into the cheese basket and place into it the salted curd, fold the cloth over the curd then add the follower and press overnight with 15 kilo of weight (I use weightlifting weights to press the cheese)

The following day peel the muslin cloth from the cheese and sit the cheddar cheese in the fridge to form a rind on a cake cooling rack. This cheese is a very long-lasting cheese and if it is waxed, it can easily be kept up to six months to mature.

For a cheese press you will need a top and a bottom plate with holes drilled in the bottom plate for the whey drainage. Sit this in a tray to catch the whey from the pressed cheese curd. Two cheese baskets, one to line with muslin and filled with the milled and salted cheese curd, then another cheese basket placed on top as a follower. Place the top plate on top of the follower, secure four dowels in place then add some weights or a large pot filled with water. Press overnight and the next morning place in the fridge to form a rind. Wax the cheese for longer keeping and maturing. The cheese can be eaten after 4–6 weeks as a mild cheddar.

Yoghurt

It cannot be emphasised enough how important it is to have good bowel flora. This is the final stage of digested food prior to evacuation from the body. It is also the place where partly digested, fermenting food particles reside. Often due to the lack of fibre in our modern diets, this mass hangs around a lot longer than is appropriate. We carry old rubbish within us without realising it and disease can build up as a result. A pale complexion, sluggishness and a general lack of vitality are outward symptoms.

Turning milk into yoghurt is an excellent way of enhancing the nutrient availability of the milk and for introducing the beneficial bacteria into the gut flora. Yoghurt is also an effective way of keeping the milk palatable for longer without refrigeration. The bacteria in yoghurt are different from that of kefir so they are two very different cultured milk products. Traditional yoghurt is not as thick as the commercial yoghurt which may have gelatins, skim milk powder and other thickening agents and additives. Most yoghurts are highly sugared even some of the so-called natural ones.

Bulgarian yoghurt is usually consumed plain and the strains used are Lactobacillus bulgaricus and Streptococcus thermophilis. This style of yoghurt is often strained by hanging in a cloth for a few hours to reduce the whey content. The resulting yoghurt is creamier, richer and milder in taste because of the increased fat ratio.

Greek full cream yoghurt is made with milk that is blended with extra cream and is often served with honey, walnuts or fruit preserves.

You will find many variations with yoghurt styles.

The most important aspect of yoghurt is the contribution it makes to our health. All the bacteria used to make yoghurt are of different types that are beneficial for our good health, but most of these bacteria do not survive the digestive tract. They are eventually killed by the digestive processes as they work their way down the gut. There are however two strains that do survive the digestive process and continue to proliferate down into the intestinal tract and take up residence in the lower bowel. These two bacteria types are ABT or acidophillis and bifidus bacteria, and ABY has lactobacillis bulgaricus added to it. This third bacteria adds a little bit of a tangy flavour and it is my favourite yoghurt. Acidophillis and bifidus are very important to us as we are born with a good supply of them, but we tend to lose them with our modern lifestyles. Antibiotics, stress and fast food all contribute to the demise of these very important bacteria.

With the regular consumption of this yoghurt, we can be assured that we have good inner health. Various yoghurt cultures can be purchased along with the cheese-making bacteria.

Making Yoghurt

Making your own yoghurt is easy:

1. Heat the milk to 80°C then allow to cool to room temperature or to 43°C

2. Incubate the yoghurt at around 43°C overnight

A little yoghurt from a previous batch can be introduced into a new batch to make yoghurt, but ... the best yoghurt to make will be from a yoghurt culture.

- Make sure the utensils are all very clean. Glass is highly recommended
- Heat about a litre of milk in a stainless-steel saucepan to 80°C
- Add two grains of the yoghurt culture to the milk when it has cooled to 43°C or below
- Set the incubator at 43°C and place the jar inside. You can also bring the milk to 43°C and pour into a thermos bottle. There are many types of yoghurt makers on the market, and they should all do the job of keeping the milk at a temperature overnight to turn it into yoghurt
- If you want a nice smooth yoghurt, you can put it through a strainer then pour the yoghurt in glass jars and place in the fridge. The yoghurt will become a little thicker upon cooling

It is also important to consume both yoghurt and kefir whilst they are still fresh.

This has to do with the lactic acid in which the (+) or right-handed form predominates, whereas the older yoghurt the (-) or left-handed form predominates. The form (+) of lactic acid in yoghurt is most beneficial to the human organism while the (-) form may have adverse effects.

Kefir

What is Kefir?

Kefir is a cultured, enzyme-rich food filled with friendly micro-organisms and yeasts that help balance our inner eco-system. Kefir also supplies complete protein, essential minerals and valuable B vitamins.

Description of Kefir

Kefir has a uniform creamy consistency, a sour, refreshing taste with a mild aroma resembling fresh yeast. Kefir also has a slight hint of natural effervescent zesty tang. There are approximately forty aromatic compounds which contribute to the unique flavour with a distinctive pleasant aroma of kefir, along with a small percentage of alcohol (.08 to 2% alcohol) while 0.5% alcohol is considered the standard result of a 24-hour ferment. This is because there are yeasts present in the kefir that can ferment the milk sugars. The yoghurt making process has a bacterial conversion while the kefir grain has both bacterial and yeast actions.

The Kefir Grains

There are two main varieties of kefir, and these are milk based and the water/sugar based grains. There is a difference between the two. The milk-based kefir, the original kefir grain that has the bacteria present to break down the milk protein, Lb. Kefiranofaciens is lost when converted to a water/sugar-based ferment. The kefiranofaciens bacteria need the milk proteins to survive and will consequently die outside of a milk environment. These bacteria are not easily re-instated, and it may take up to two months of 48-hour culturing in fresh, raw milk to re-activate it if it does at all. The kefir grain that has no kefiranofaciens bacteria may still thicken the milk on culturing, but the kefir grain itself won't expand itself anymore.

The de-hydrated form of kefir that you find commercially available apparently does not have that important bacteria in it and cannot be classified as a true kefir grain. If you're in doubt about the originality of your kefir grains, you can see if your kefir culture is a true kefir (with all the right bacteria and yeasts in place) when the grains multiply themselves with subsequent batches.

The true milk-based kefir grains

are a curd of gelatinous white biomass. This bio matrix has 13 Lactobacilli, 5 Streptococci/ lactococci bacteria and 7 types of yeast. This wonderful combination of micro-organisms has a powerhouse effect on our intestinal flora thus contributing greatly to an enhanced immune system and therefore vital good health. Kefir is easily digested and cleanses the intestines of toxic waste and provides vitamins, minerals and complete proteins. Kefir can contribute greatly to the well-being of AIDS sufferers and sufferers of chronic fatigue syndrome, herpes and cancer. It also has a tranquillising effect on the nervous system. The regular use of kefir can help relieve all intestinal disorders, promote bowel movement, reduce flatulence and create a healthier digestive system. Apparently, kefir can also help eliminate unhealthy food cravings by making the body more nourished and balanced.

The water/sugar kefir

looks more translucent and has a dense feel due to the constant pressure of the carbon-dioxide gas that is the by-product of an alcoholic ferment. There are many other beneficial bacteria and yeasts that contribute to bowel health, so it is worth considering this type of kefir ferment. Dried or fresh herbs can also be added in the kefir ferment. When transferring milk kefir grains to a water-based ferment there will be a time lag of three to four days whilst the organisms cease to reproduce while they fatten up by storing energy with the different forms of sugar in their environment.

After the third batch or so, the grains will have fully adjusted to their new food medium and will do their job in 48-hour batches. When the traditional milk-kefir grain has been changed to a water-based ferment, it will not successfully revert to its former state as Lb.kefiranofaciens. You may have a successful-looking ferment but it will be without the fighting power of the missing microbe that can inhibit the growth of coliform and other fecal bacteria, C.albicans and even cholera.

Anti-tumour properties are also attributed to the traditional kefir grain.

How to Make Kefir

Making your own kefir is so simple.

1. Take a clean glass jar and fill with milk.
2. Place the kefir culture in it and screw a lid on the jar and stand at room temperature for twelve to thirty-six hours depending on ambient room temperature.
3. Strain or fish out the kefir grain before consuming it.

That's all!

Having said this, books are written on this fascinating and health promoting food. Let's take a closer look at the finer art of making kefir and how to fine-tune the process.

- A slightly warmer than ambient temperature will speed up the fermentation process.
- Using more kefir grains in the milk will speed up the fermenting process
- Don't leave the ferment out too long before refrigerating it as it will turn too sour to enjoy
- Keep the kefir out of direct sunlight
- A glass a day is a recommended amount or as much as you feel comfortable   with
- Some kefired milk from one batch to another is ok to kick-start the fermenting   process
- It is not recommended to rinse your kefir grains between batches as active bacteria are present on the surface of the grains that are otherwise lost down the sink
- Use fresh and preferably raw milk but any milk will do
- Always have very clean utensils when making kefir to avoid contamination
- Use more rather than fewer kefir grains in the milk to avoid contamination

How to Use Kefir

Use kefir to ferment cream into sour cream
Use kefir to ferment cream and make butter
Use kefir to ferment milk and make a light curd cheese
Use kefir milk in smoothies mixed with fruit, nuts etc

Storing the kefir grain

There are times when kefir isn't part of your daily routine, and the grains need to be kept viable. Storing kefir is a simple process of placing the grain in a clean jar in fresh milk and placing it immediately in the fridge. This will provide food for the organisms for several weeks. It would be kind to the kefir grains to remember them every now and then and say good day to them with a fresh batch of milk. They will thank you for it. If for some reason the jar works its way to the back of the fridge where it becomes forgotten, it is possible to revive the kefir grains after a couple of months of neglect by culturing and re-culturing them for several batches until the resulting kefir grain becomes healthy again. Kefir grains can also be frozen. It is important to defrost them slowly in the fridge otherwise they will die.

Sour cream

To ferment cream, take some kefired milk and add a few tablespoons to some fresh cream. The cream can be raw or pasteurised as the pasteurised cream will come back to life with all those organisms found in the kefir. Keep the jar on the bench until the thick cream turns solid and there are signs of fermentation. This can be seen by the airholes through the glass jar. It has long-lasting qualities and can be kept for months in the fridge. It simply becomes thicker and richer with time. Whip it up when very cold, until it becomes a stiff cream for serving with sweet or savoury dishes.

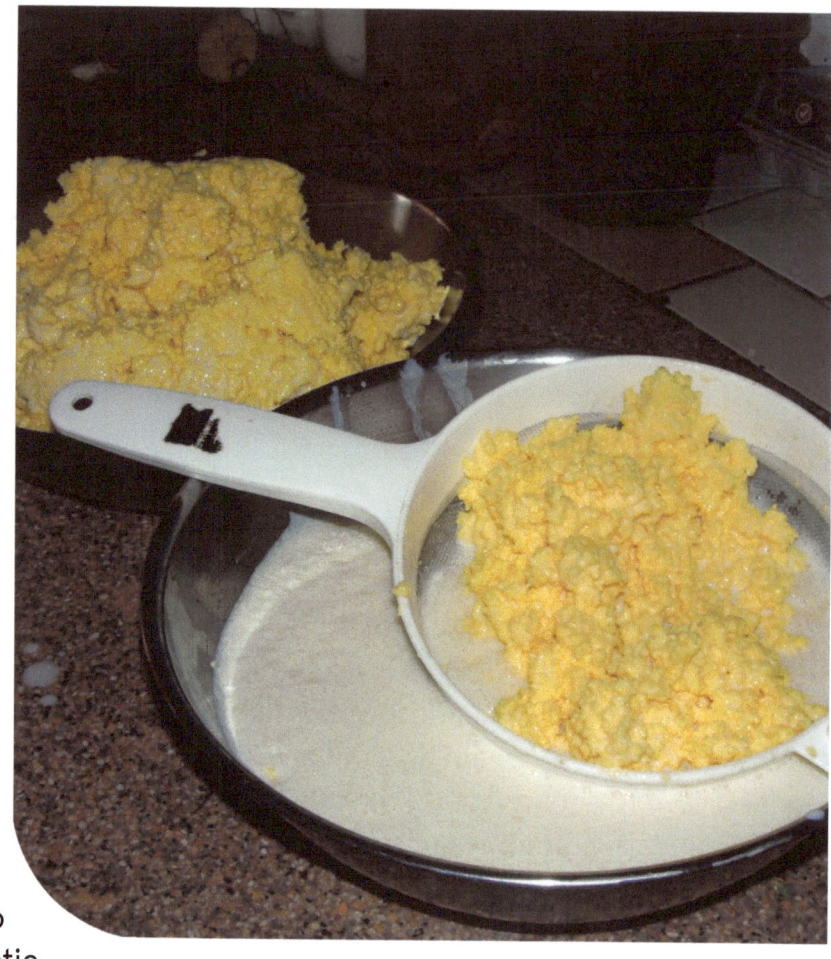

Cultured Butter

Cold fermented sour-cream can easily be turned into butter, and this then becomes fermented or cultured butter. Making butter is quickly done in the food processor and making it this way takes much less time than using fresh cream. Strain off the buttermilk then the butter will need to be washed three times or until the water runs clear. The butter is then squeezed as much as possible to drain any water. No salt is needed as the butter has lactic bacteria in it due to the fermentation process. This gives the butter longer lasting keeping qualities and can easily be kept outside the fridge for easy spreading on your bread. The butter tastes great, and it has a stronger taste than butter made with fresh cream.

Another method of fermenting cream for making cultured butter:

If you can source your cream from an organic cow, you can simply leave the cream out of the fridge for 24–48 hours. The cream will spontaneously ferment as the lactobaccilis bulgaricus bacteria that are naturally found in the cow, will induce a ferment that pre-digests the fats and the proteins and sets the cream solid. Place the cold fermented cream in the food processor and wiz until butter has formed. If you are not sure when it has completely formed into butter, watch for the butter to clump around the blade and see that the buttermilk has totally separated from the yellow butter grains.

Cultured Butter

1. Place the cold fermented cream into the food processor

2. Whiz until the cream turns to butter

3. Strain the butter from the buttermilk

4. Wash the butter at least three times in cold water or until the water runs clear

5. Work the excess water out with a wooden spoon or with your hands and place the butter in containers. Butter can be frozen for many months.

Butter made this way does not need the addition of salt as the lactic bacteria that is present in the butter will help to preserve it a lot longer than sweet butter. The added advantage is that it can be kept outside the fridge even in the summer.

The resulting buttermilk is also a very healthy and beneficial drink. Until I learnt of the benefits of yoghurt I enjoyed a daily glass of buttermilk.

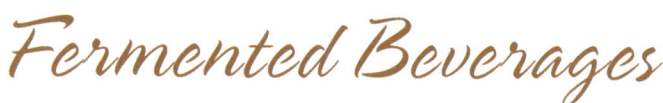

Fermented Beverages

Cereal grains can present difficulties with phytates and the assimilation of their nutrients, but by fermenting them into nutritional thin gruels they become valuable additions to the daily diet. Fermented drinks have been a part of every culture and often the peasant would bring his traditional brew along into the field as a liquid meal and thirst quencher. This liquid mini meal helps to give the field worker extra stamina to keep him at his daily labour. These beverages are more thirst quenching than plain water due to the addition of minerals and usually these ferments have a very low amount of alcohol. If this is a problem, you can add sour whey or an equivalent and this will take care of the yeasts that are working on the sugars as the sugars become lactic acid instead. These drinks are very nutritious and easy to assimilate.

The following are some lacto-fermented beverages from around the world:

Bousa from Egypt – an opaque drink made of wheat, and Boza – a traditional Turkish beverage made by yeast and lactic acid bacteria fermentation of millet, cooked maize, wheat, or rice semolina/flour. Boza in Albania is made of maize and wheat flour, sugar and water. It has a sweet-to-sour taste.

Chicha from South America is a clear, bubbly beverage made with corn. Balls of cooked corn mush are chewed and inoculated with saliva, then added to water and allowed to ferment. The taste is similar to kombucha.

Kiesel from Russia and Poland is an important grain-based lacto-fermented drink made from stale rye bread.

Kombucha from Russia is made from tea, sugar and a mushroom culture.

Kvass from Russia and the Ukraine is a lacto-fermented drink usually made from stale rye bread or beetroot.

Munkoyo from Africa is a lacto-fermented brew, containing less than 0.5 percent alcohol, made from millet or sorghum. Also called sorghum beer, it is consumed in large quantities by field workers and at celebrations. It is also given to babies to protect them against infection and diarrhoea.

Pulque is from Mexico and is a lacto-fermented drink made from the juice of the agave cactus. With time, it goes alcoholic. Distilled pulque is tequila.

Fermented Rice Milk

This recipe comes from Egypt. Fermented grain drinks are traditionally prescribed for nursing mothers, but anyone will gain extra strength and stamina through them.

I have extended the fermenting time of the traditional recipe, and it improves the flavour.

½ cup rice (white or brown)

8 cups of water

1 teaspoon sea salt

2 tablespoons sour whey/ water kefir

Honey

Cinnamon

1. Cook the rice in water for long enough for the rice to become soft and mushy
2. Cool the rice and liquid then whiz through a food processor or a blender
3. Pour into a large jar and add 2 litres of water with salt and whey/water kefir
4. Place the lid on tight and sit on the bench at room temperature for several days and taste for a slightly soured flavour
5. Add honey and cinnamon as desired

All traditional fermented gruel drinks are based on much the same recipe as the fermented rice drink. Feel free to experiment with other grains

Rejuvelac

This very simple drink can be made from wheat, spelt or rye grains. It is rich in lactic-forming bacteria and all the goodness from the grains including live enzymes, minerals and vitamins will add to the nutritional benefits of this living thirst quencher.

Half a cup of sprouted grains will make 4 cups of rejuvelac.

1. Sprout the grain in a large glass jar covered with a Chux or muslin cloth held by an elastic band. Soak in water for 12 hours then turn the bottle upside down to drain the water out.

2. Turn the bottle back up and allow the grains to sprout until the little tails just begin to form.

3. Add the 4 cups of water and leave to soak for 1–2 days depending on ambient temperature. At this stage there will be some activity evident with some fizz. Pour the water into a bottle and keep in the fridge where it will keep up to a week.

4. You can reuse the sprouted grains for another batch, and it will take only 24 hours of soaking next time.

Ginger Beer

Ginger roots are rich in yeasts and lactic acid bacteria, and made into a ginger bug, it will become active quickly. You can also use turmeric and galangal, but they all need to be organic or fresh so that the microbes are still intact. If it comes from overseas, they have most likely been irradiated and not alive with yeasts and microbes.

The ginger bug starter

1½ cups water

3 teaspoons finely chopped or grated ginger root

3 teaspoons sugar

Glass jar

Butter muslin or open weave cloth and an elastic band

1. Fill the glass jar three quarters full of warm water
2. Add the sugar and ginger
3. Cover with the cloth and elastic band to keep it in place

Feed the bug starter every day for seven days with 1 teaspoon of sugar and 1 teaspoon of chopped or grated ginger. Stir twice daily and after a week you should see activity with fizzing and bubbling. It will also take on a mild yeast-like smell and become cloudy in colour. You are now ready to make the ginger beer. If not using the starter bug immediately, feed it every other day for a few days. Otherwise, refrigerate it and feed 1 tablespoon of ginger and sugar weekly. To reactivate it, take it back to room temperature and begin feeding it again.

Ginger Beer

3 cups sugar

2 teaspoons cream of tartar

1 litre boiling water and 5 litres cold water

2 lemons juiced and strained

1. In a large bowl or bucket add the sugar and cream of tartar then pour in the boiling litre of water

2. Stir to dissolve the sugar before adding the cold water

3. Pour in all the liquid of the ginger beer starter bug

4. Add the strained lemon juice

5. Stir well and then pour into six 750 ml bottles. It is recommended that you use plastic soft drink bottles as ginger beer is inclined to explode, especially in hot weather

6. Store in a cool, dark place for two weeks before drinking. Carefully open the lid to allow the air to escape and hold over the kitchen sink

Restore your ginger beer starter bug:

→ Take the jar with the left-over solids and fill with water to the top.
→ Tip out half or give to a friend so that they can make their own starter bug.
→ Fill back up three quarters full of warm water and feed for another week.

Lactic Fermented Ginger Ale

1 small piece of ginger about 2 cubic centimetres, very finely grated

Juice of one lemon, strained

¼ cup honey

½ teaspoon sea salt

2 tablespoon sour whey/ water kefir

1 litre water

1. Mix everything thoroughly in an airtight container, and let it sit at room temperature for 3–7 days.

2. Strain the ginger ale and pour into flip top bottles or plastic soft drink bottles.

3. Refrigerate once it's fully carbonated.

Lacto-fermented ginger ale mixed with kombucha tea is a great thirst quencher.

Water Kefir

Water kefir grains, also known as sugar kefir grains and they are a culture of bacteria and yeast held in a complex symbiotic relationship. The true water kefir is different to the milk kefir that has been turned into a water-based kefir as they come from two different sources. The true water kefir has its origins from the cactus plant. Water kefir is found all around the world with no two cultures being the same. Water kefir, like the milk kefir, has a wide mix of over forty different strains of healthy bacteria and yeasts. There are dozens of vitamins, minerals, nutrients and enzymes that water kefir provides, and when used as a probiotic and refreshing drink, it will produce a carbonated beverage for everyone to enjoy. Water kefir is one of the easiest ways to improve your overall health and digestion and the grains can be easily purchased online.

How to ferment the water kefir

½ cup of sugar

2 litres water

½ teaspoon organic molasses

4 tablespoons water kefir grains

1. Stir the sugar, molasses and kefir grains into the water in a wide-mouth glass jar until dissolved.

2. Leave the grains to ferment at room temperature for 24 hours or more

A traditional drink made in Mexico is water kefir with pineapple, brown sugar and cinnamon.

Coconut milk can be incubated with a couple of tablespoons of water kefir grains. Try it after 24 hours. It can thicken the coconut milk to make a cultured coconut cream. Doing this too often will weaken the kefir grains though

NB   add a little organic molasses only every 5 or 6 batches to give the water kefir grains the minerals they need. Feeding molasses too often will overwhelm them.

Water Kefir Soft Drink

1. Make a batch of water kefir and strain out the liquid

2. Combine 1/3 of water kefir with 2/3 of fruit/ vegetable juices

3. Don't fill right up to the top of the bottle but rather leave some room for the gas to build up

4. Culture 24–72 hours at room temperature before refrigerating

   Carefully open the bottle as it can have quite some fizz

Take caution as the water kefir can turn the fruit juice into alcohol if left longer after it feel tight with gas. Leaving a bottle in a hot car and drinking it will get you into real trouble!

Orange-Ginger Carrot Kvass

Kvass is commonly made from either bread or beets, but it might be an acquired taste for most people. This recipe turns it into an effervescent beverage with carrots, ginger, and orange. It is tangy, fragrant and pleasant to drink. A second fermentation with a bit of sweetener added gives it quite a fizz.

6 carrots thinly sliced

2 tablespoons roughly chopped ginger

6 large strips of organic orange peel (peeled with a vegetable peeler)

teaspoons sea salt

¼ cup sour whey/ water kefir

1. Put carrots, ginger, and orange peel into a two-litre glass jar. Add salt and whey/ kefir and fill the remainder of the jar with water. Stir well to dissolve in the salt.

2. Cover the jar with a clean cloth or muslin. Secure with an elastic band and place in a warm spot to ferment for 2–3 days depending on ambient room temperature

3. Strain the liquid from the carrots, leaving about 1 cup of liquid in the jar for another round of kvass

4. A second fermentation can now be made to give it a vibrant fizziness

5. Place the kvass in flip top bottles with a pinch of sugar or honey for a little bit of sweetness and added carbonation

6. Allow to ferment for 1–3 days depending on the ambient room temperature

NB: To make a second but weaker batch of the first ferment, simply add more water to the leftover one cup of liquid from the first batch with two added teaspoons of sea salt. Repeat the fermentation.

Lactic-Fermented Sweet Potato Fly

Sweet potato fly is not unlike a ginger ale. It has a sweet, tangy and spicy flavour and you may like to try this unusual beverage.

2 large, sweet potatoes	1 teaspoon nutmeg
2 cups of sugar	½ teaspoon ginger
½ cup of sour whey/ water kefir	1 eggshell, cleaned and crushed
2 lemons juiced and zested	4 litres water
2 teaspoons cinnamon	Coarsely grate the sweet potatoes

1. Rinse into a strainer to get rid of the starch (you may like to save the sweet potato starch and use it for cooking purposes)

2. Combine the grated sweet potatoes with all the other ingredients in a fermenting bucket, glass or plastic container

3. Stir, cover, and allow to ferment at room temperature for around three days or until fermented enough

4. Strain through a fine sieve lined with an open-weave cloth and bottle into airtight bottles. Refrigerate and serve

Kombucha Tea

This ferment is a paradox as a health beverage: how can black tea and white sugar turn into a liver cleansing drink? Kombucha is created by a mushroom/ scoby that floats on top of the tea and with the tannins and sugar combination ferments the tea and creates a myriad of compounds that contribute greatly to our good health.

There is an amazing list of what the kombucha mushroom has in store for us:

- Acetic, lactic acid, glucuronic acids, enzymes, vitamins, carbonic acid, caprylic acid, citric acid, oxalic acid, usnic acid, vitamins B1, B2, B3, B6 and B12 and C, folic acid, amino acids, and other substances with antibiotic, antiseptic and detoxifying characteristics are all formed within this fermented tea.
- Kombucha also contains polyphenols, electrolytes, minerals, organic and amino acids, billions of probiotic bacteria such as bifidus, enzymes that help to rejuvenate, replenish, regenerate, recharge, rebuild, and balance the body.
- Kombucha is known to be helpful in cases of inflammatory arthritis because of its detoxifying effects on the liver.
- Tannins are broken down to about a half of regular tea. Tannins are needed by the scoby to impart its nutrients and benefits into the tea
- Sugar is converted into acids, resulting in a sour taste when no sugar remains
- The pH is naturally balanced with kombucha and it also helps to cleanse and remove damp and toxins from the body
- Kombucha tea also helps to improve digestion and assists the spleen in the delivery of more nutrients

The scoby transforms sweetened black tea into a slightly fizzy sour drink,

These all work together to help the body recover its natural healing ability.

Most commercial tea is very high in fluoride so it is highly advisable that you use organic tea so it will contain only a very small amount of fluoride.

3 litres of water

180 gram of white or raw sugar (white sugar seems to work the best)

2-3 tablespoons of black loose-leaf tea or 5 tea bags.

One large piece of kombucha mushroom plus some tea from a previous batch.

1. Make up the tea, add the sugar and cool to room temperature.

2. Place the scoby into the cold tea with some tea from a previous batch and leave to ferment for at least 10–14 days.

There are two basic methods to make the tea: batch method and continuous method. I prefer the continuous method as it's much less work. I always have two batches on the go, and they are sitting on the bench in a couple of crock pots with a small dispenser tap at the bottom. I found the crock pots at the local tip shop for $1 each and they are the base for the 10-litre spring water bottles from a local water supplier. When one batch of tea gets down towards the bottom, I will brew up a big kettle of tea, add the sugar, cool it to room temperature and pour it into the crock. In a week or so I will be able to drink from it again whilst taking from the other one until it gets used and so on. There is no need to worry about contamination as the tea usually ends up a bit too acidic for drinking after a while, especially in the hot summer months. The acidity will keep any pathogens at bay, and I just add some more sugar to the crock to make it more palatable to drink.

The new mushroom that will eventually grow on top of the mother is the scoby for the next batch of tea. Give the original mother to a friend to make their own refreshing kombucha tea.

A second ferment can be made the same way as the water kefir soft drink. This usually takes around ten days to develop the fizz.

Beet Kvass

The humble beetroot has a whole host of minerals, vitamins, antioxidants and anti-cancer properties. The anti-inflammatory molecules from betaine found in beets may show cardiovascular benefits, and the betalin pigments in beetroot supports the second phase of detoxification where broken down toxins are bound to other molecules so they can be excreted from the body. Beetroot is also known to purify the blood and the liver.

Turning beetroot into a lactic fermented drink gives us a wonderful tonic and healing tool. It can be used for chronic fatigue, chemical sensitivities, allergies and digestive problems. When assembling the beet kvass, use more rather than less beetroot to make it a thicker and sweeter drink as beetroot is full of natural sugars.

1. Cut two to three medium size beetroots into coarse cubes and place them in 1 litre of water

2. Add 1 level teaspoon of sea salt and 2 tablespoons of sour whey/ water kefir

3. Leave to stand at room temperature for around 10 days or until it has a slightly sour taste

4. Skim off any white mould that floats on top as this can taint the kvass

5. Store in the fridge for up to several months

Bon appetit!